FOUR SEASONS

Movement

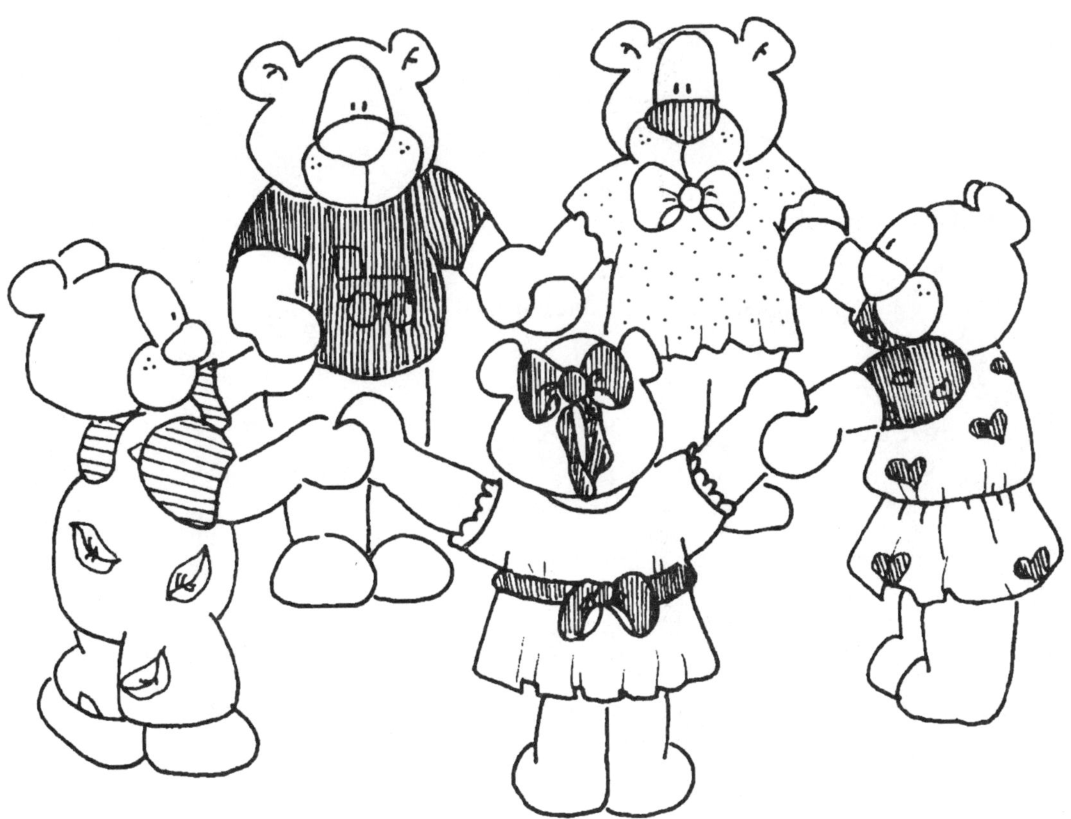

By Jean Warren

Illustrated by Marion Hopping Ekberg

Formerly Titled ***Movement Time*** *by Monday Morning*

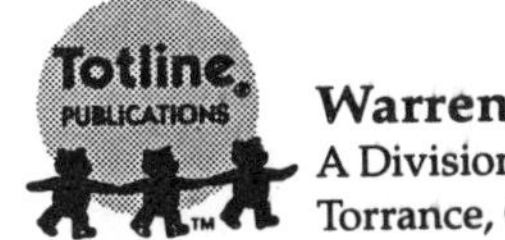

Warren Publishing House
A Division of Frank Schaffer Publications, Inc.
Torrance, California

To the Potter Family: John, Margaret, Josh, Jordan, Jared, and especially Megan—MHE

Managing Editor: Kathleen Cubley
Editor: Gayle Bittinger
Contributing Editors: Susan Hodges, Elizabeth McKinnon
Copyeditor: Mae Rhodes
Proofreader: Kris Fulsaas
Editorial Assistant: Suzi Butler
Book Design/Layout: Sarah Ness, Carol DeBolt
Cover Design: Brenda Mann Harrison
Production Manager: Jo Anna Brock

ISBN: 1-57029-090-3

Library of Congress Catalog Card Number 95-62117
Printed in the United States of America
Published by: Totline® Publications

Editorial Office: P.O. Box 2250
Everett, WA 98203

Business Office: 23740 Hawthorne Blvd.
Torrance, CA 90505

20 19 18 17 16 15 14 13 12 11 10 9 8 7 6 5 4

Introduction

As young children grow and develop, they need many opportunities to express themselves. Through open-ended movement activities, children can explore their feelings, interpret visual suggestions, and experiment with their own solutions to hypothetical problems.

Four Seasons Movement provides parents and teachers with a collection of practical ideas that are developmentally geared to young children. As they participate in the activities, children will discover the relationship between their bodies and the space they move in. They will practice a variety of movement skills, such as hopping, rolling, and throwing, and explore movement concepts, such as fast and slow, high and low, and backward and forward.

The activities are designed to exercise children's imaginations as well as their bodies. Individual ideas are grouped by theme under appropriate seasonal headings. Each group includes a creative warm-up exercise and one or more songs or poems to be accompanied by movements. There might also be a story or an imaginative situation for which your children are asked to perform the actions or make up their own endings or solutions. Or there may be an activity that encourages the children to practice observations and coordination skills as they move in ways analogous to animals and things in the world around them, such as caterpillars or machines.

Adults should be enthusiastic when they are presenting a movement idea to young children, but they should also be prepared to abandon an activity if the children become disinterested. Although some of the activities are more structured, most leave the action to the children's willingness and imagination. It is best to let the performers decide which story elements should be acted out and to accept their interpretations, however bizarre. The more freely children are encouraged to express themselves through their body movements, the more confident they will become in communicating their ideas in general.

Contents

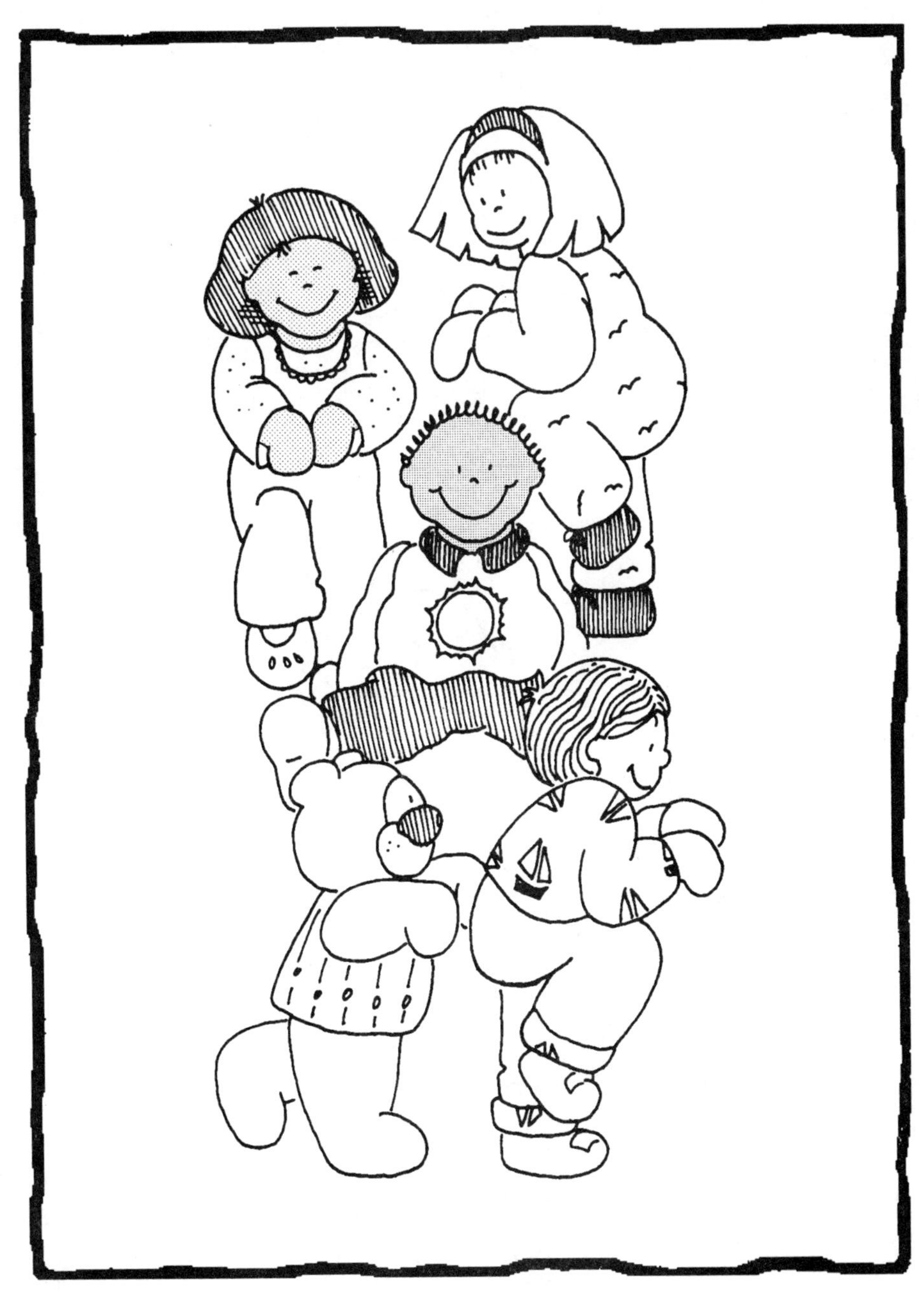

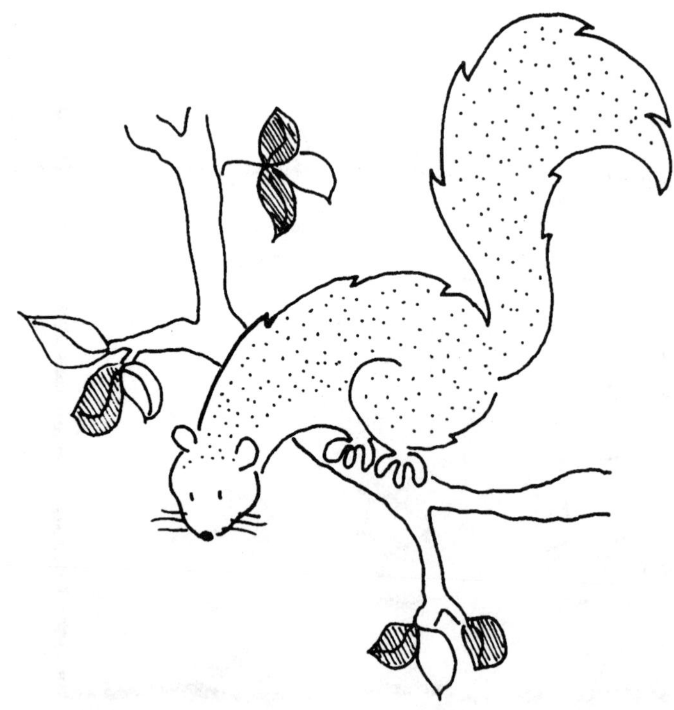

Fall

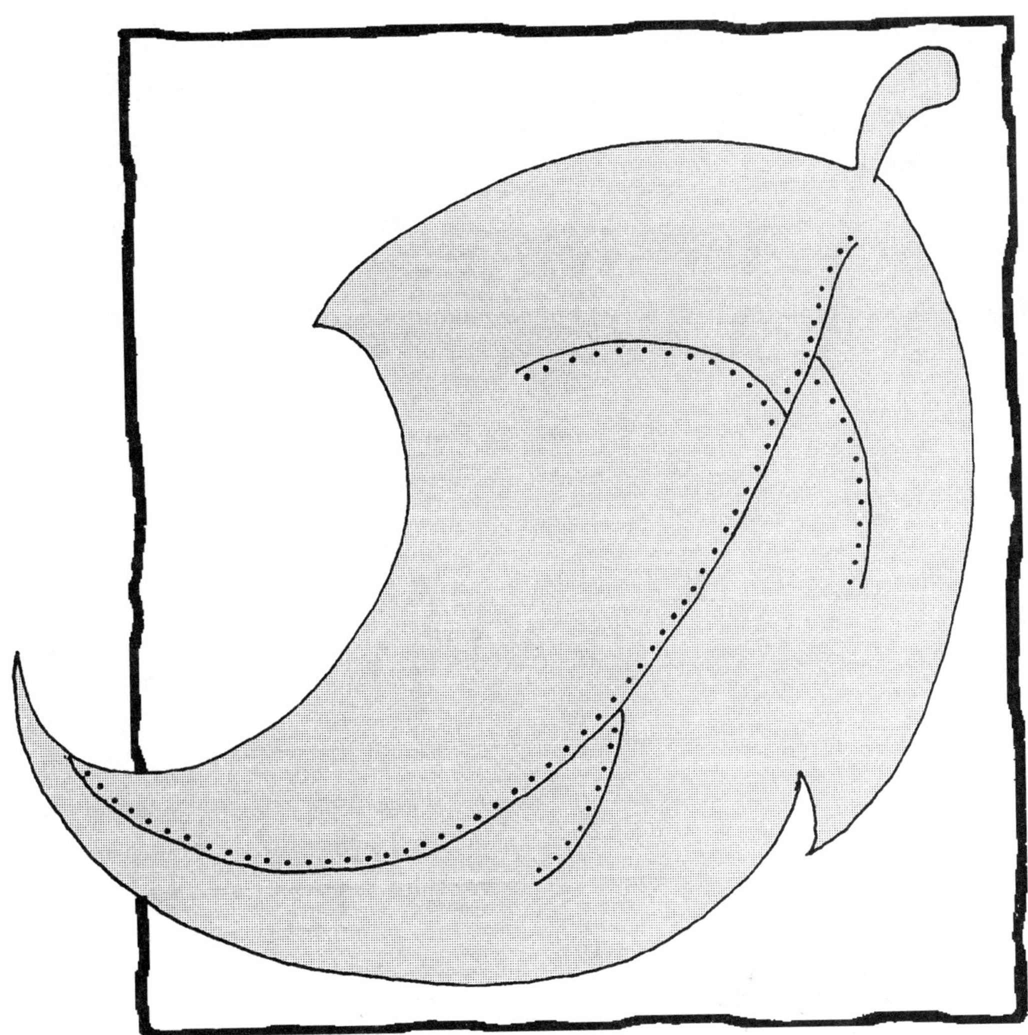

Handy Warm-Up

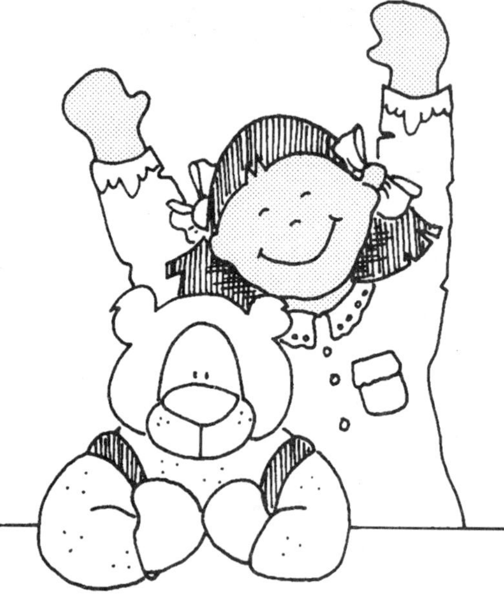

Have your children hold their hands still while they examine them. What do their hands look like? Now have the children see how far out, up, and down they can stretch their hands. Use the following ideas to help your children experiment with finding different ways to move their hands, fingers, and wrists.

- Pretend to place a large, heavy box in front of each child. Have the children pretend to pick up their boxes and lift them over their heads.
- Let your children pretend to pass around something slimy, something sticky, or something round.
- Ask your children to show you gentle hands, rough hands, weak hands, strong hands, working hands, and playful hands.

Harvesting Movements

As you finish the general warm-up exercises above, move into more specific ways hands can be used to harvest fruits and vegetables. Ask your children to climb an imaginary ladder and use their hands to pick fruit such as apples, oranges, and cherries. Next have the harvesters climb down from their ladders and dig in the dirt with their hands to gather potatoes and pull carrots. Let your children name other fruits and vegetables for everyone to "harvest."

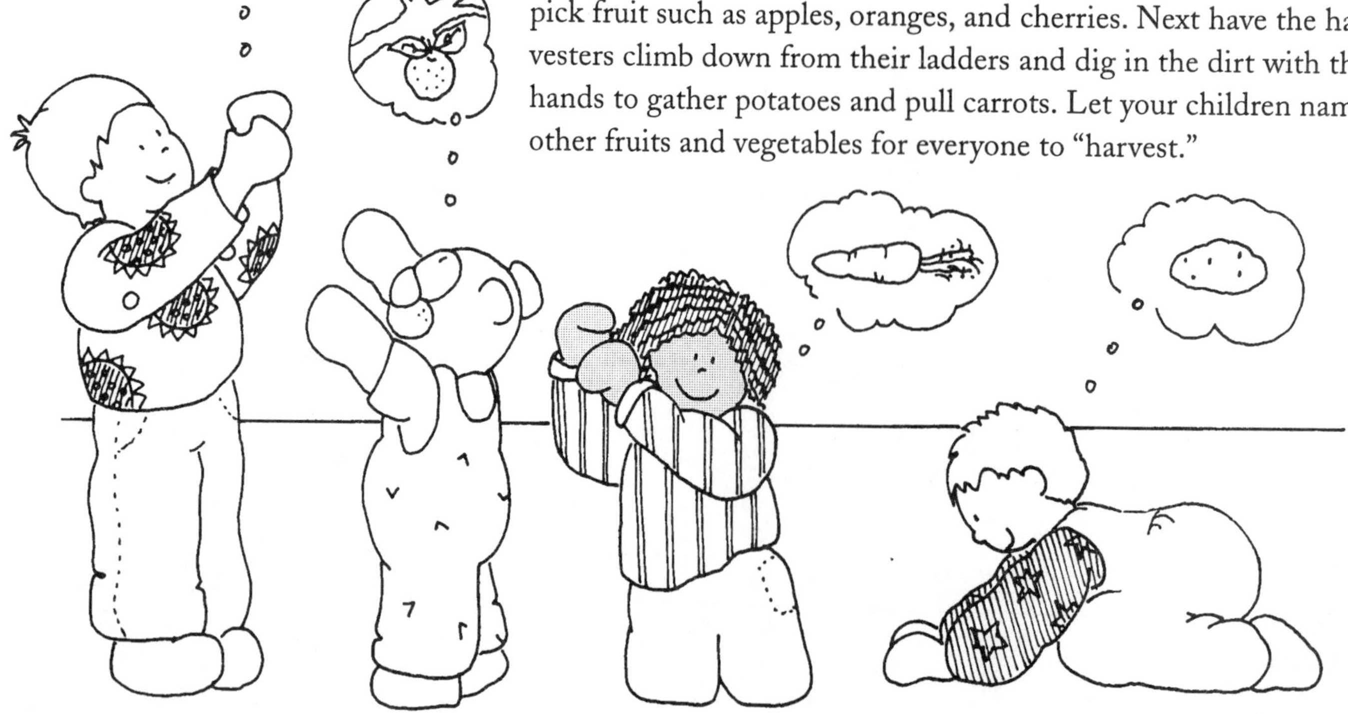

Vegetable Soup

After your children have harvested all their fruits and vegetables, ask them to help make some Vegetable Soup. Have everyone stand around an imaginary soup pot, stirring as they add the vegetables. Let your children decide which vegetables to add to the pot. As they stir, sing the following song.

Sung to: "The Farmer in the Dell"

The soup is boiling up,
The soup is boiling up.
Stir slow, around we go,
The soup is boiling up.

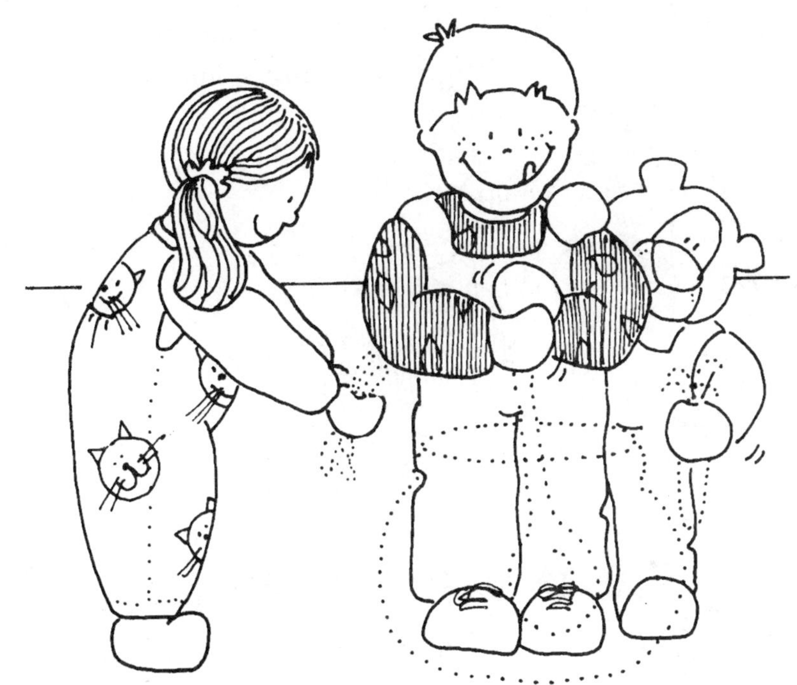

First we cook the broth,
First we cook the broth.
Stir slow, around we go,
First we cook the broth.

Now we add some carrots,
Now we add some carrots.
Stir slow, around we go,
Now we add some carrots.

Continue with additional verses about other vegetables your children would like to add to the soup. Finish with the following verse.

The soup is ready now,
The soup is ready now.
Stir slow, around we go,
The soup is ready now.

Jean Warren

Pretend to serve a bowl of soup to each child. Encourage your children to "eat" the delicious soup they made together.

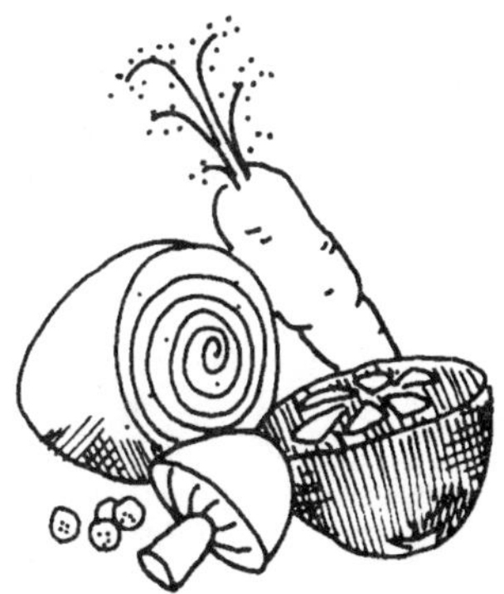

Leafy Warm-Up

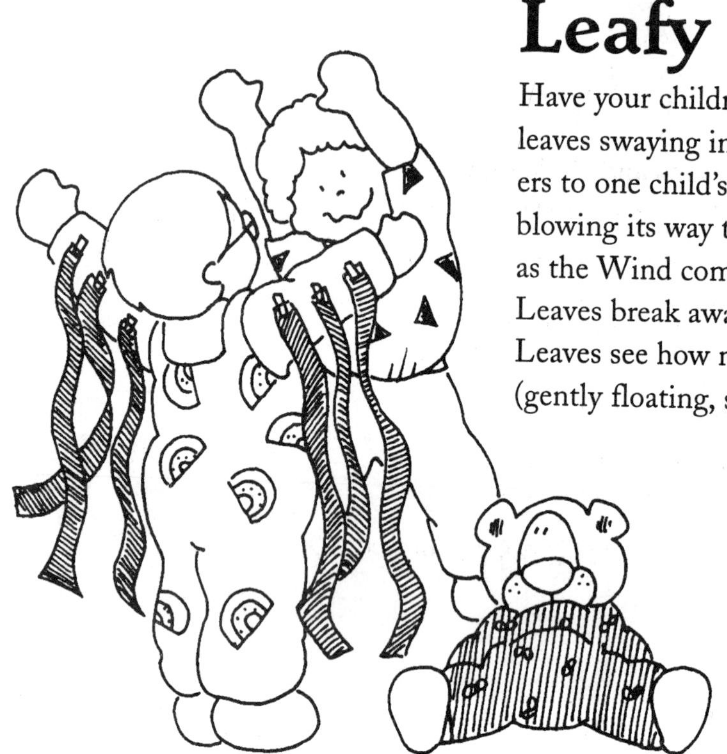

Have your children imagine that they are beautifully colored autumn leaves swaying in the autumn breeze. Tape long crepe-paper streamers to one child's arms and have that child pretend to be the Wind, blowing its way through the Leaves. Have the Leaves begin to flutter as the Wind comes closer. When the Wind blows hard, have the Leaves break away from the tree and fall to the ground. Let the Leaves see how many different ways they can fall to the ground (gently floating, spinning, swaying, bouncing, and so on).

☆ Raking Leaves

Ask your children to pretend that they are out raking autumn leaves. Have them rake all the leaves into a large pile. When the leaves are all together, choose one of the following endings to act out (or let the children choose).

- Let your children play in the leaves—rolling in them, sliding on them, or tossing them into the air.
- Have your children wear streamers on their arms and pretend to be the wind, scattering the leaves all over.
- Divide the children into pairs. Have one child in each pair pretend to be a giant bag, holding his or her arms open in a wide circle. Let the other child in the pair pick up armfuls of leaves and stuff them into the "bag."

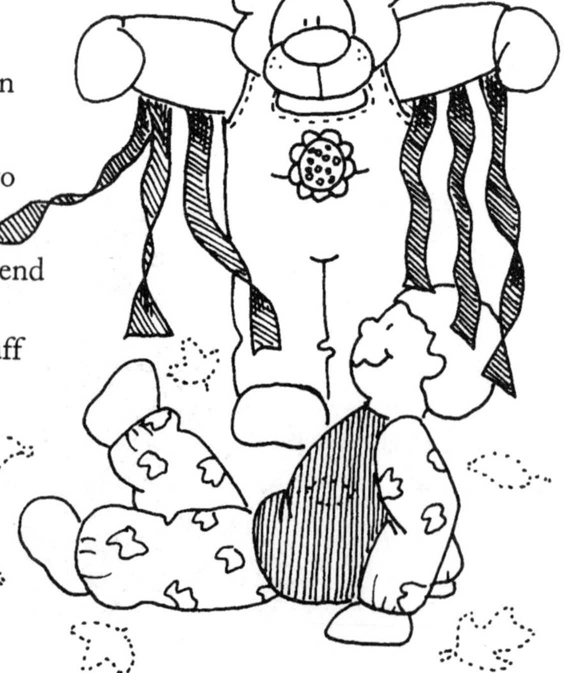

Falling Leaves

Sung to: "Twinkle, Twinkle, Little Star"

All join hands and circle round
(Hold hands and walk around in a circle.)

While we watch the leaves fall down.

See them skipping here and there,
(Stop and make hands move like leaves.)

Dipping, flipping in the air.

All join hands and circle round
(Hold hands and walk around in a circle.)

While we watch the leaves fall down.

All join hands and circle round
(Hold hands and walk around in a circle.)

While we watch the leaves fall down.

Autumn leaves so peacefully
(Stop and gracefully float hands to ground.)

Falling, falling from the tree.

All join hands and circle round
(Hold hands and walk around in a circle.)

While we watch the leaves fall down.

Jean Warren

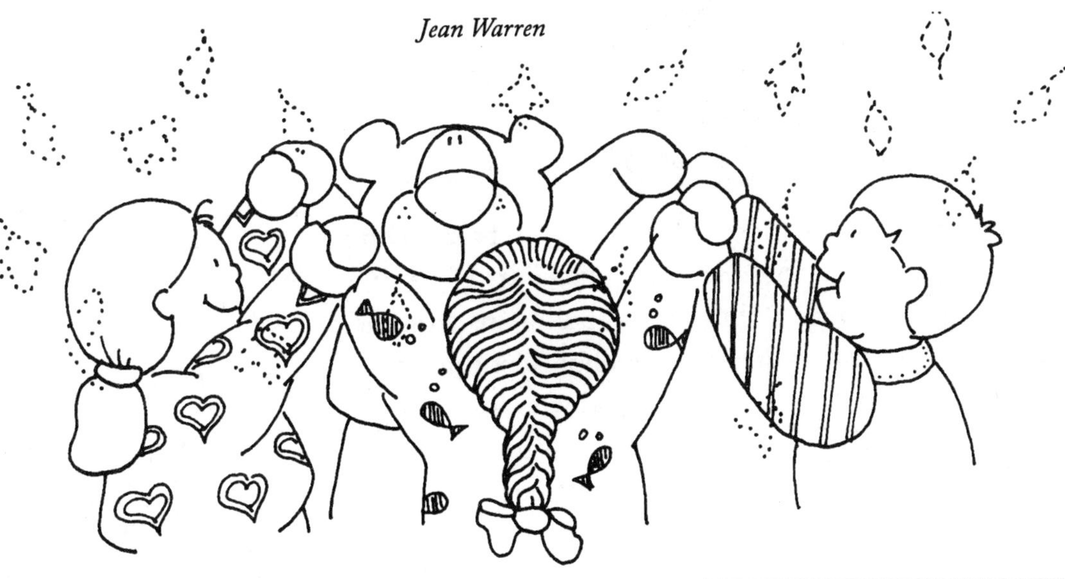

Down, Down

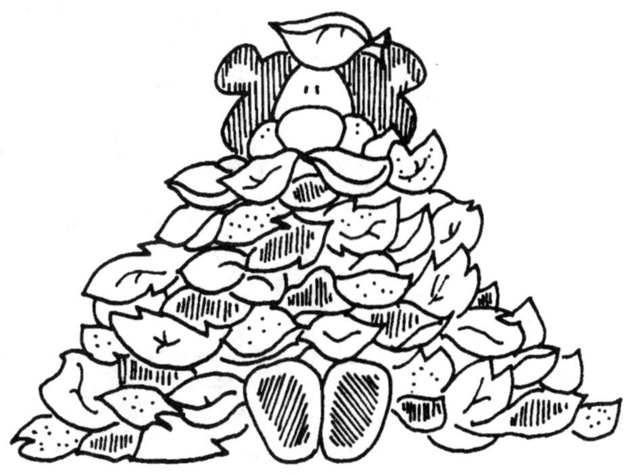

Down, down, yellow and brown,
(Flutter fingers down to the ground.)

Fall the leaves all over the ground.

Rake them up in a pile so high,
(Pretend to rake leaves.)

They almost reach up to the sky.
(Reach arms up and stand on tiptoes.)

Adapted Traditional

Cat Warm-Up

Explore the characteristics of cats with your children. Ask them to imitate cat movements and show you how cats walk, play with a ball of string, curl up in front of a warm fire, or show that they are angry or afraid. Let this activity be a lead-in to the following dramatization about a black cat on Halloween.

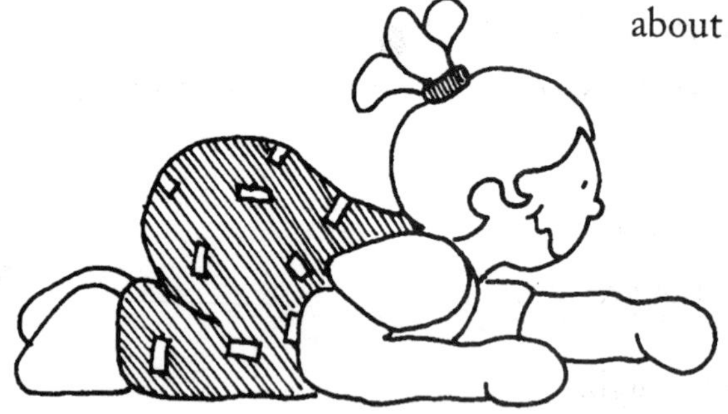

Halloween Story

A little black cat is slinking about lost, cold, hungry, and scared on a Halloween night. What things might have frightened it? Have your children act out scary Halloween sights, such as pumpkins with their glowing grins or trick-or-treaters dressed as goblins. Continue the story by telling the children about a friendly child who finds the lost cat, brings it home, lets it dry out by the fire, feeds it some doughnuts, and makes a bed for it. Encourage them to act out each part of the story as you tell it.

Variation: Let your children develop and finish the story themselves—it will probably have a more imaginative ending!

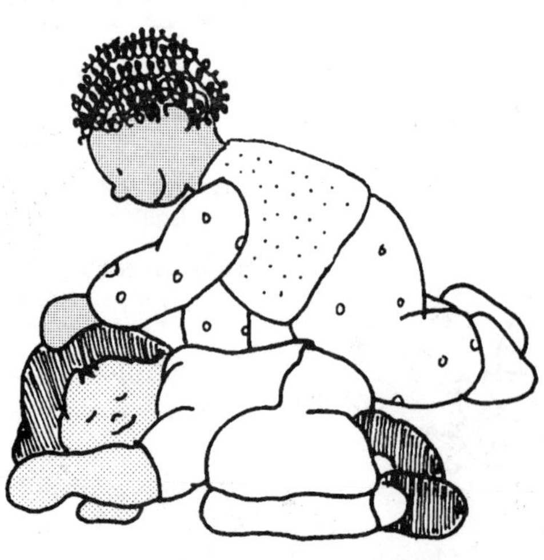

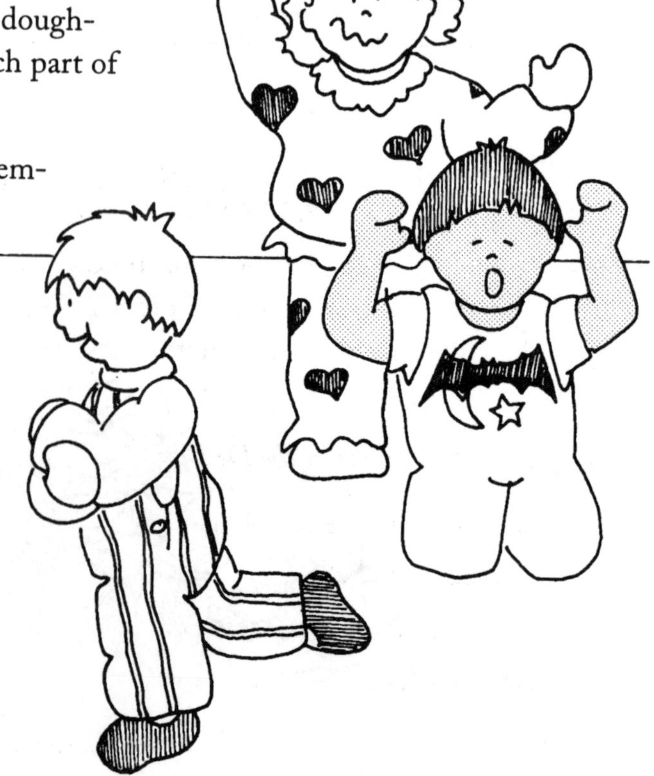

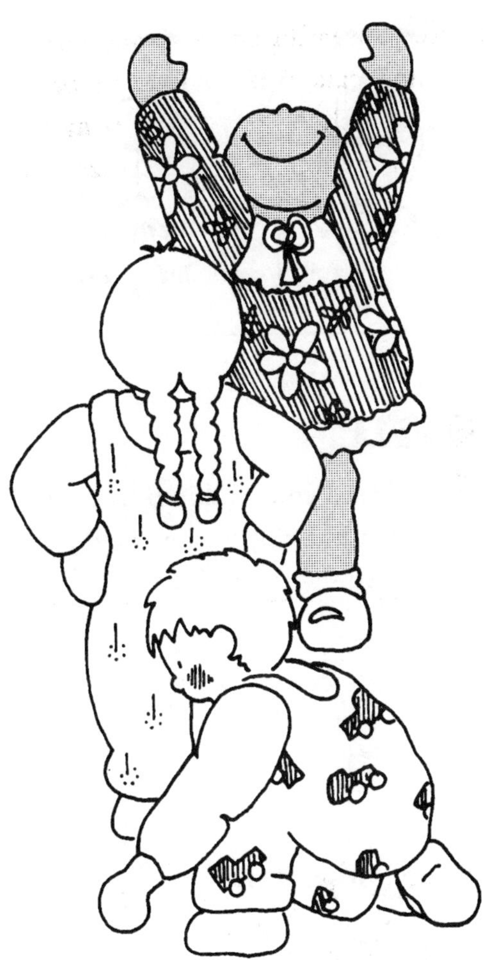

Black Cat

Have your children pretend to be black cats as you read the following poem. Ask them to listen carefully and do the motions as they are described. If you wish, you may substitute the name of any other Halloween character, such as *white ghost, pumpkin, scarecrow,* or *spider,* for *black cat.*

Black cat, black cat, turn around.
Black cat, black cat, touch the ground.

Black cat, black cat, jump up high.
Black cat, black cat, touch the sky.

Black cat, black cat, reach down low.
Black cat, black cat, touch your toe.

Adapted Traditional

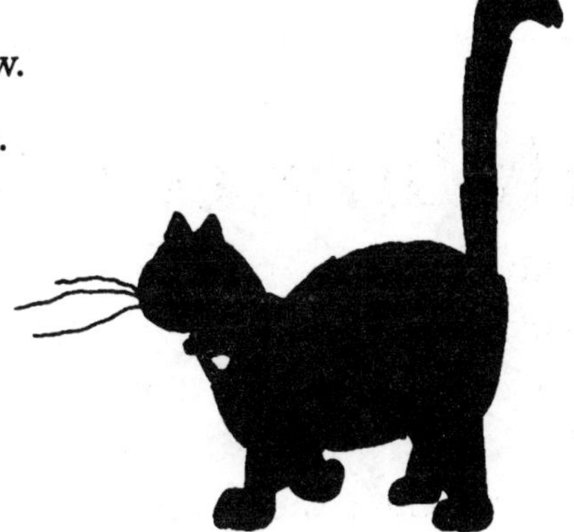

See the Black Cat

Place a piece of string on the floor in a straight line. Tell your children that the string is the top of a fence. Sing the following song and have the children act out the motions as indicated. When it is time to "walk across the fence," have them walk carefully along the string.

Sung to: "The Farmer in the Dell"

See the black cat run,
See the black cat crawl.
See the black cat walk the fence,
It doesn't even fall.

Jean Warren

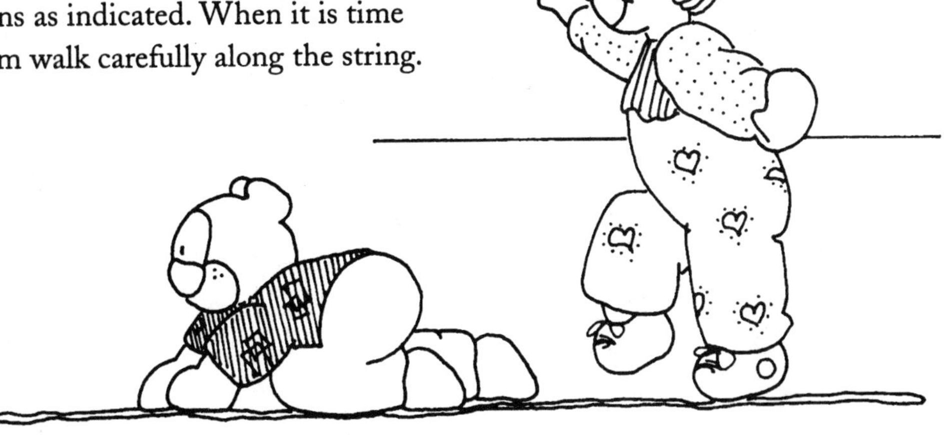

Owl Warm-Up

Have your children sit in a circle and pretend to be owls. Explain to them that owls stay very still and often only move their eyes and head. Ask them to look at various objects around the room, moving only their eyes or their head to do so. Then, one at a time, ask each "owl" to fly around the room and find a pretend tree to perch on. Continue with the following activity.

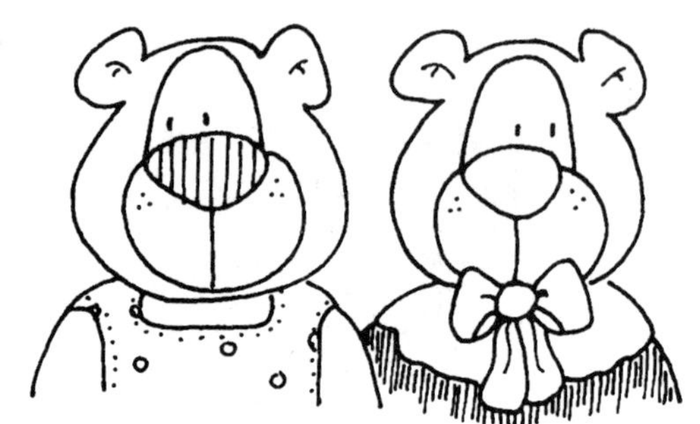

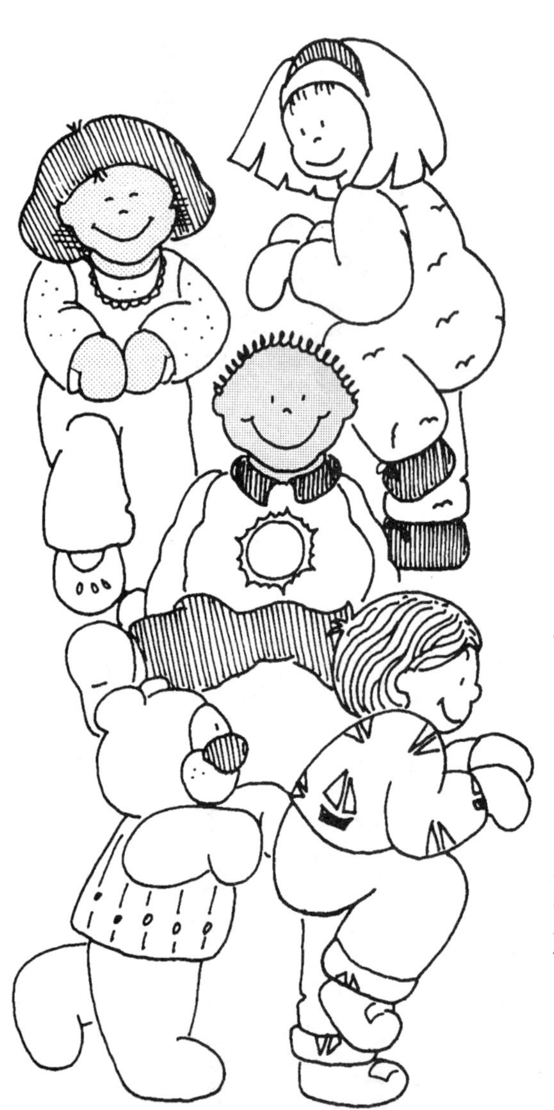

Wise Owl Game

Begin with the warm-up activity above. Have your children fly back to the circle. Select one child to sit in the middle of the circle and be the Wise Owl. Help the rest of the children say the following.

Wise owl, wise owl
Sitting in the tree,
Wise owl, wise owl,
What do you see?

Help the Wise Owl respond with the following verse.

I see cats
Running by me
All night long
As I sit in my tree.

Jean Warren

When the Wise Owl says the name of an animal, have the rest of the children pretend to become this animal and move about the room accordingly. Let the Wise Owl choose another child to take his or her place. Play the game again, letting the new Wise Owl choose another animal to substitute for *cat.* Continue the game until everyone has had a chance to be the Wise Owl.

The Wise Old Owl

As you tell this school version of the folktale "Too Much Noise," let your children act out the motions and make the sounds.

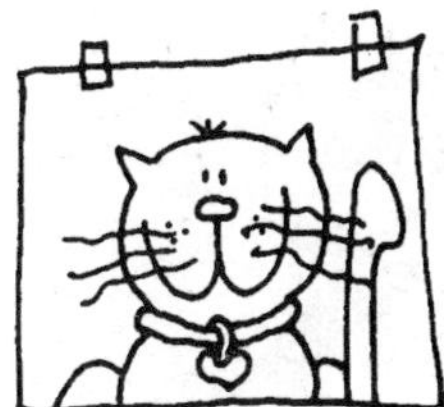

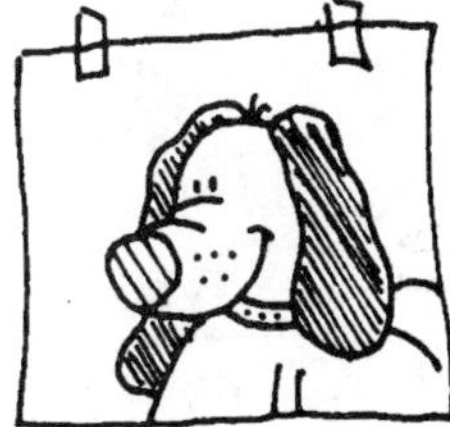

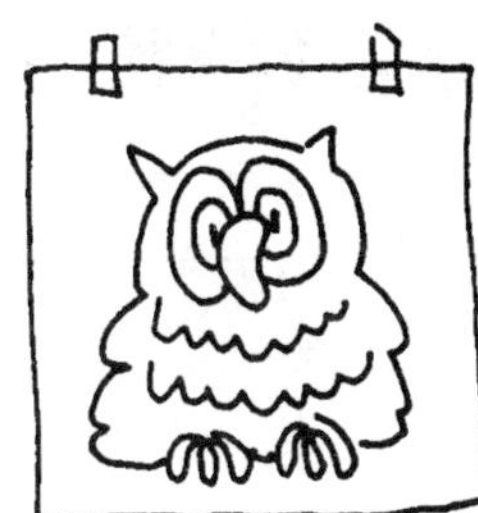

"One day at school, a teacher was very unhappy. The children made too much noise when they walked *(shuffle, shuffle, shuffle)* and when they talked *(buzz, buzz, buzz).* She didn't know what to do, so she went to the Wise Old Owl, who told her to buy a cat. The next day she bought the cat and took it to her class. Now all day she heard *(shuffle, shuffle, shuffle), (buzz, buzz, buzz),* and (*meow, meow, meow).*The teacher was still unhappy, so she went back to the Wise Old Owl, who this time told her to buy a dog. The next day she bought a dog and took it to school. Now all day she heard *(shuffle, shuffle, shuffle), (buzz, buzz, buzz), (meow, meow, meow),* and *(woof, woof, woof)."*

Continue telling the story, having the Wise Old Owl advise the teacher to get a pig, a cow, and a horse. Once her classroom is filled with all those animals and is very noisy, have the Wise Old Owl tell her to get rid of them. To her surprise, once the animals are gone, her room seems so quiet. Now all she hears is the quiet shuffle of little feet *(shuffle, shuffle, shuffle)* and the quiet whispers of her children *(buzz, buzz, buzz)!*

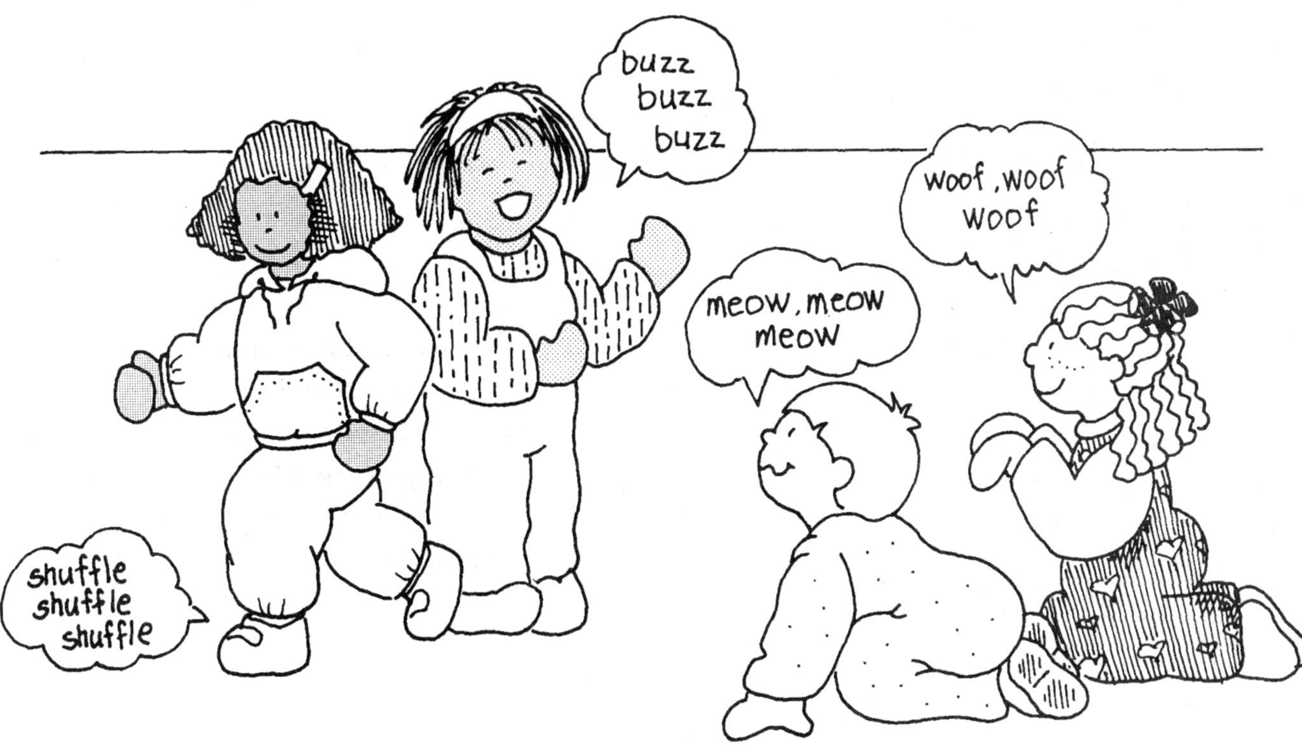

Pumpkin Warm-Up

Ask your children to join hands to form a long, winding pumpkin vine. Select every second or third child to become a pumpkin. Have the "pumpkins" crouch down low and hug their knees. At your signal, have the other children "pull" the pumpkins off the vine by gently rolling them over onto their side. Have the pumpkins roll away. Repeat until every child has had a turn being a pumpkin.

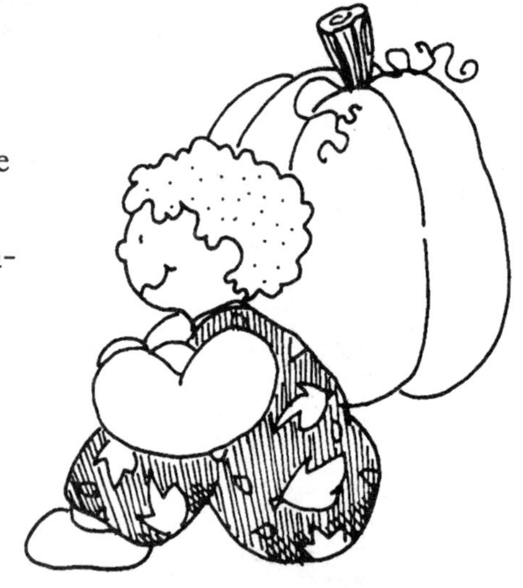

The Growing Pumpkin

After finishing the warm-up above, lead into this activity. Read the following poem. Have your children pretend to be the pumpkin seed that sprouts, grows, and eventually turns orange.

Early one morning as the sun came out,
A little white seed began to sprout.
It pushed its head up through the ground,
Waved its arms, and looked around.
At first the plant was very small,
But then the plant began to crawl.
It grew up the hill to the very top
And there, at last, it decided to stop.
Out popped a flower, a great big one,
As gold as the color of the summer sun.
The plant was happy, until one day
The beautiful flower fell away.
Then the plant grew sad, it felt real low,
Until a green ball started to grow.
It grew and grew to a great big size,
Then turned bright orange—what a surprise!

Jean Warren

See the Pumpkin

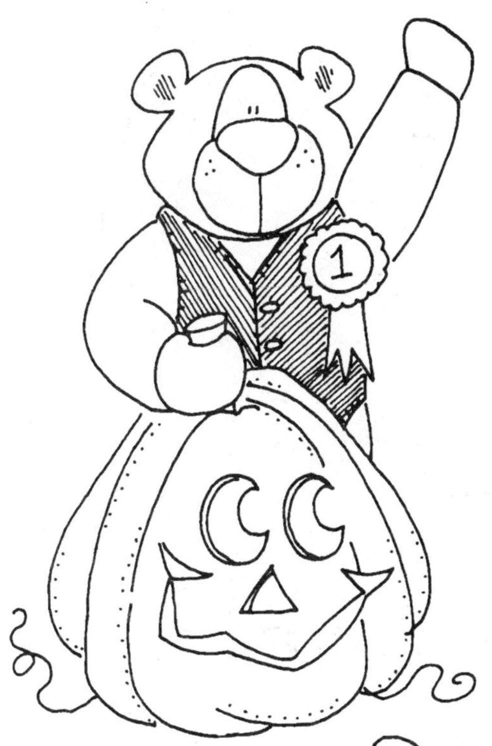

Sung to: "Did You Ever See a Lassie?"

Come and see the pumpkin,
The pumpkin, the pumpkin.
Come and see the pumpkin
We picked from the patch.
We cleaned it and carved it,
And cleaned it and carved it.
Oh, come and see the pumpkin
We picked from the patch.

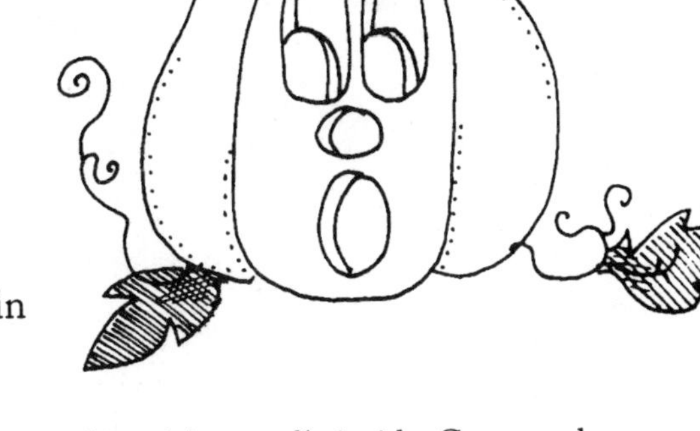

Additional verses: Come and see the pumpkin with a candle inside; Come and see the pumpkin with a big crooked grin.

Jean Warren

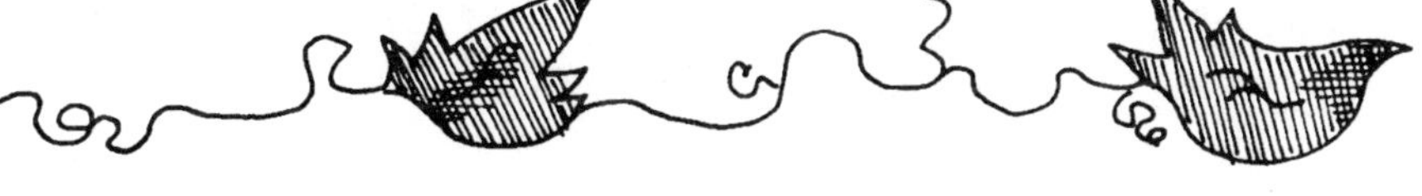

Pumpkin, Pumpkin

Pumpkin, pumpkin
Sitting on the wall,
(Sit on floor.)
Pumpkin, pumpkin,
Tip and fall.
(Fall to one side.)
Pumpkin, pumpkin
Rolling down the street,
(Roll on floor.)
Pumpkin, pumpkin,
Trick-or-treat!
(Jump up and clap.)

Author Unknown

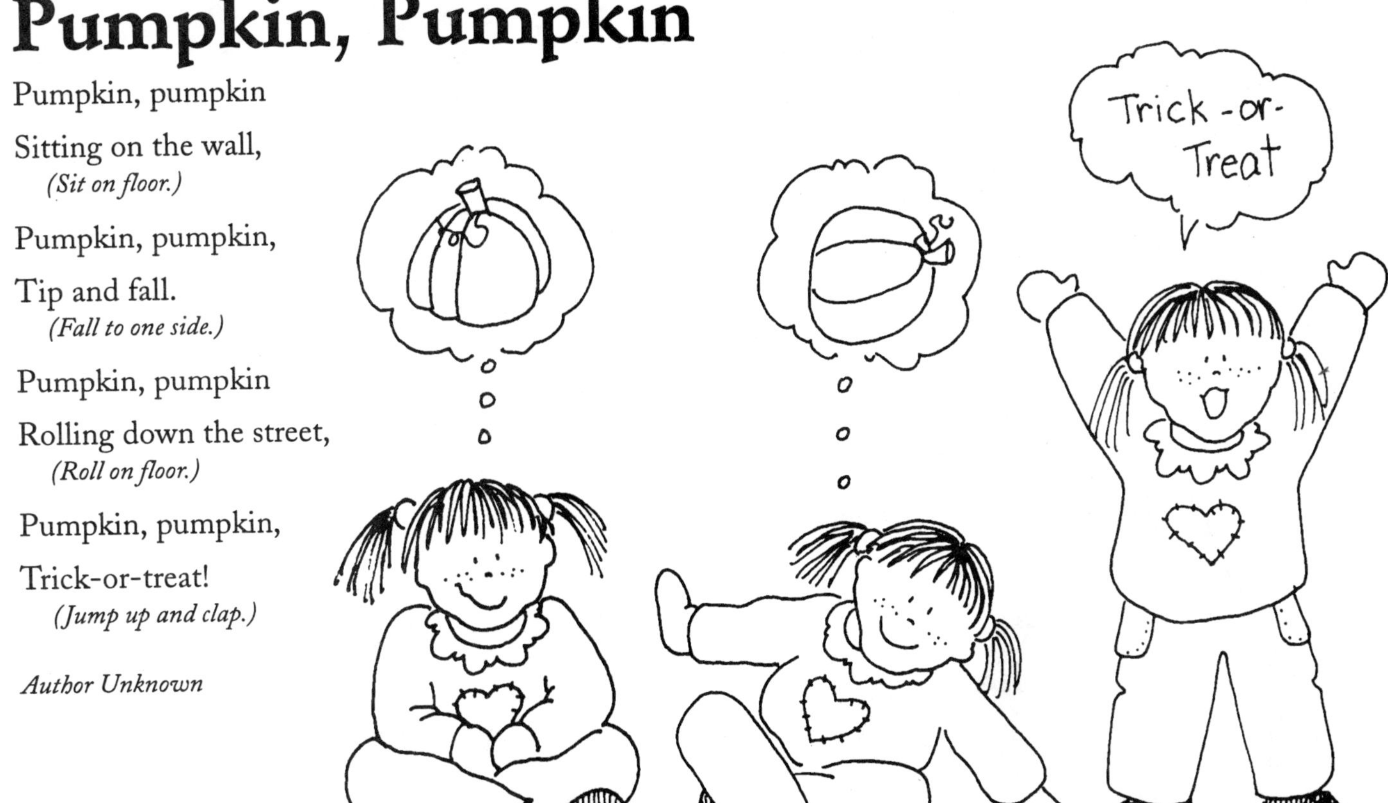

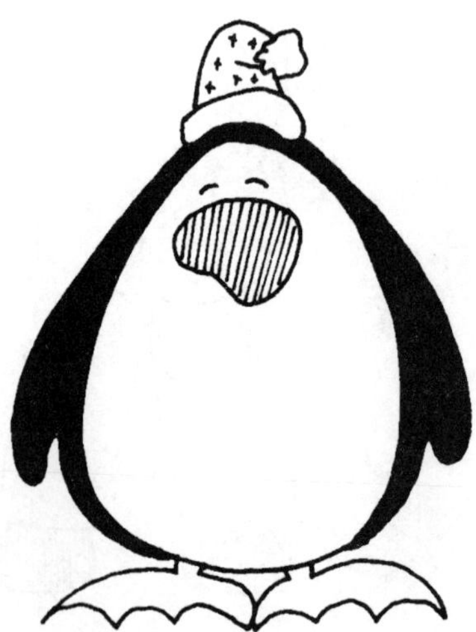

Winter

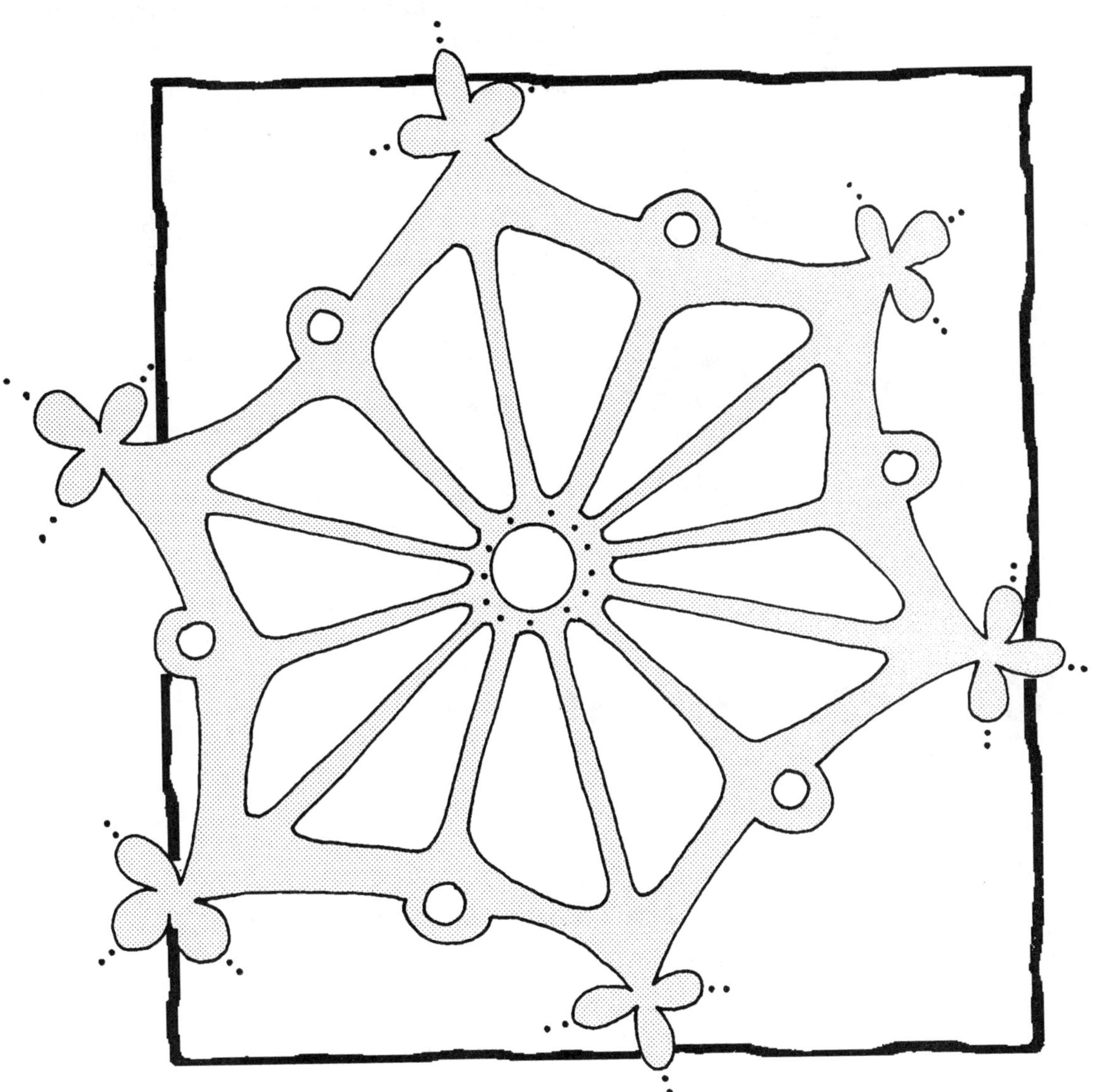

Doll Warm-Up

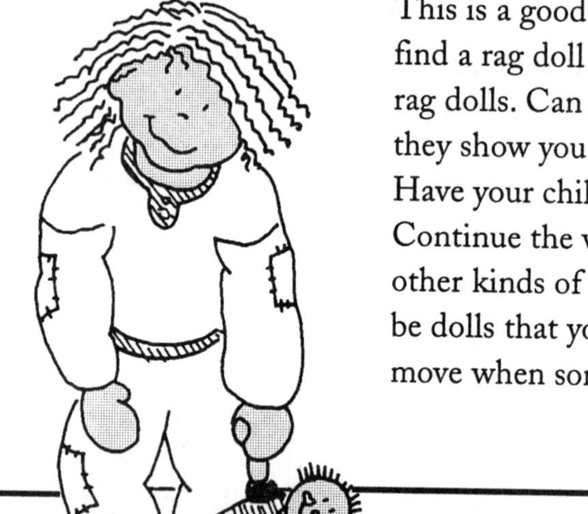

This is a good exercise for loosening up and relaxing muscles. First, find a rag doll and show it to your children. Have them pretend to be rag dolls. Can they make their bodies go limp like the doll's? Can they show you how a rag doll would move from one place to another? Have your children move each part of their body in a floppy fashion. Continue the warm-up by asking your children to show you how other kinds of dolls might move. For example, they could pretend to be dolls that you wind-up, marching dolls, or marionette dolls that move when someone pulls their strings.

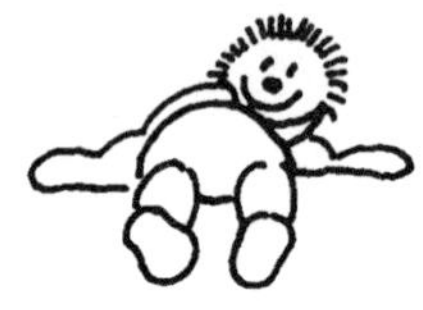

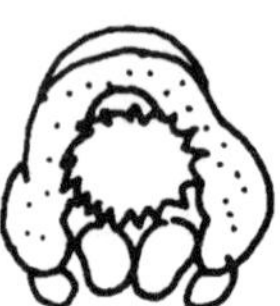

Musical Toy Story

Tell your children this holiday story. Have them pretend to be toys and sing and dance as indicated.

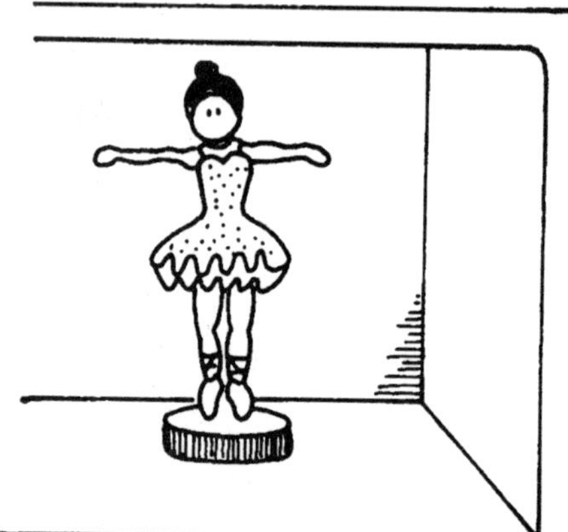

"One Christmas Eve, Santa was getting ready to pack up all his toys. Before he put them into boxes; however, he decided to test them one last time. He took a small music box out of his pocket and opened the lid. It played a little tune." (Hum the tune of "Frère Jacques.") First the music woke the ballerina doll. She got up and started to dance and sing." (Have your children dance while singing the song on the following page.)

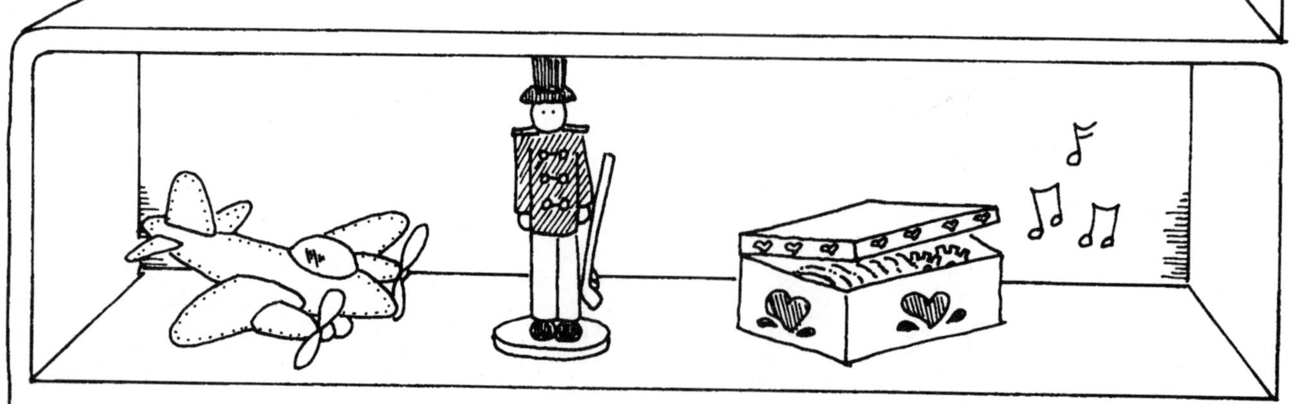

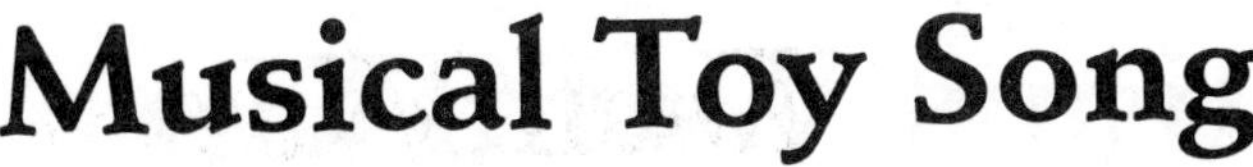

Musical Toy Song

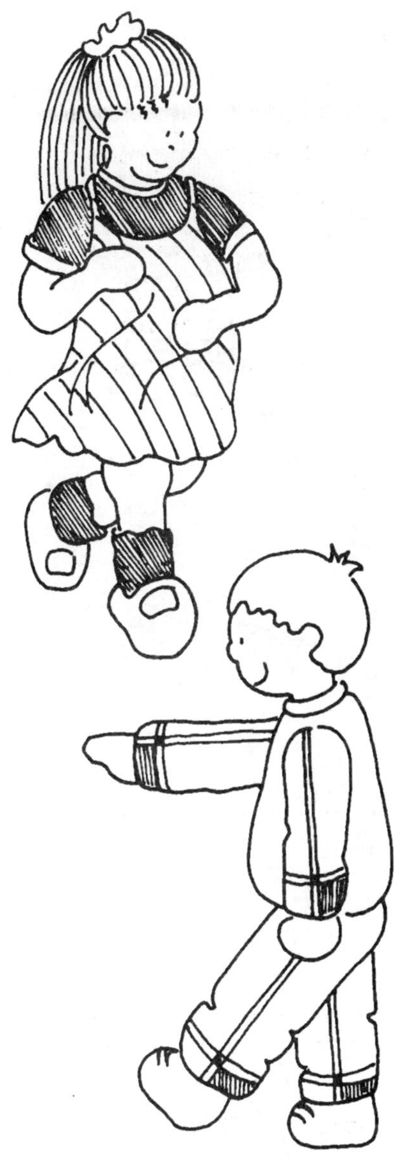

Sung to: "Frère Jacques"

I am dancing, I am dancing
Round and round, round and round.
First I turn one way,
Then I turn the other way,
Round and round, round and round.

Now continue the story from the previous page. "Santa was pleased with the way the ballerina doll danced, so he wrapped her up and put her into his sack. Next, a tin soldier got up and started marching to the music." (Have your children march while singing the next verse.)

I am marching, I am marching
In a row, watch me go.
First I march one way,
Then I march the other way,
In a row, watch me go.

"Next, the model airplane awoke, revved up its engines, and took off." (Have your children pretend to fly while singing the next verse.)

I am flying, I am flying
Round and round, up and down.
First I fly one way,
Then I fly the other way,
Round and round, up and down.

Jean Warren

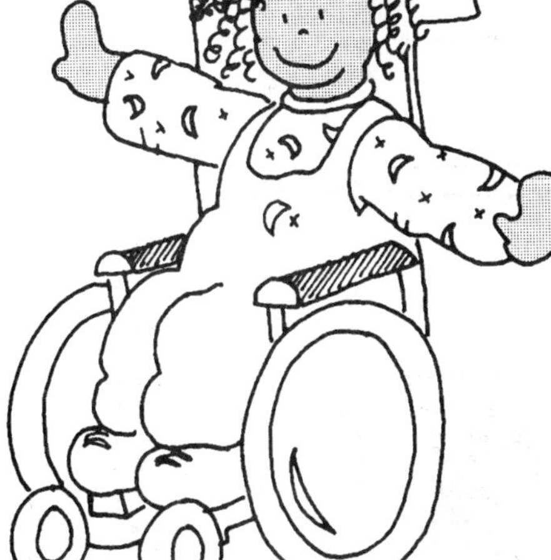

Continue with other toys and movement verses as you wish, until Santa's sack is quite full.

Decorations Warm-Up

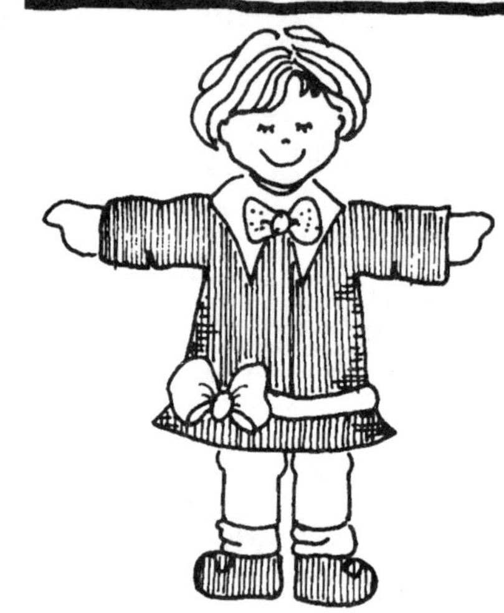

Show your children an assortment of real tree decorations, including tinsel, blinking lights, a string of popcorn, and several ornaments. Discuss the characteristics, such as the shape and texture, of each decoration. Next, pretend to decorate a tree with those few decorations. There just aren't enough and you are feeling very sad. Brighten up as you think of ways the children can help you make some more decorations.

- Ask five children to stand in a close circle. Have the children join hands in the center of the circle to make a five-pointed star. Let the children walk slowly in a circle to make the star spin.
- Have each child become a Christmas ball by rolling into a ball shape on the floor. Show the children how to fashion a hook by extending one arm and bending the hand.
- Let your children pretend to be tinsel. Have them stand tall and straight as if they were in the box. Then, have them float to the ground as they are gently tossed onto the tree. Also show them how to bend at the waist and and let their arms hang straight down as if they were draped over a branch.
- Have the children pretend to be twinkling lights on the Christmas tree by spreading their arms to make the wires and blinking their eyes for the light bulbs.
- Pretend to make popcorn in a giant skillet. Pour in some oil and have the children jump in and curl up like small kernels of corn. Turn on the heat and have the "kernels" squirm and wiggle as the pan gets hot. Have them roll every which way as they get hotter and hotter. Finally, have them jump up with a loud "pop!" When the popcorn is all popped, line up the fluffy pieces and string them together to make a garland for your tree. Have the children join hands to string the popcorn, then wrap themselves around an imaginary tree by moving in a spiral.

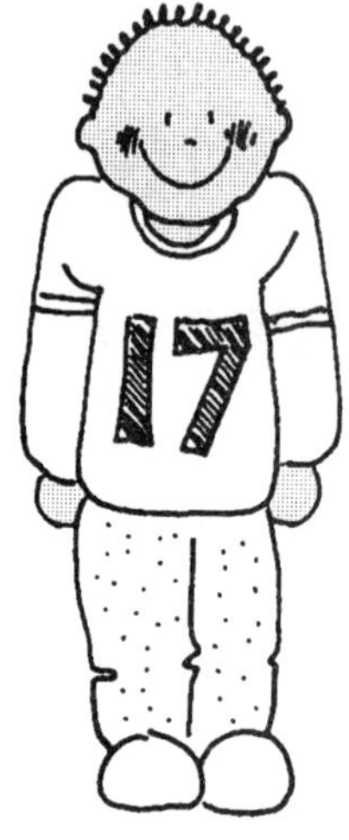

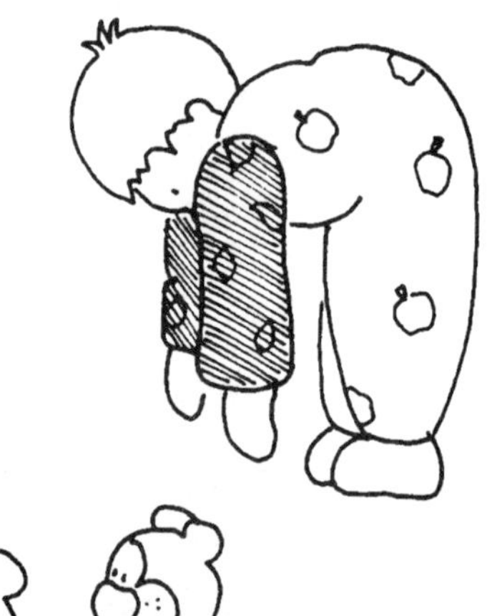

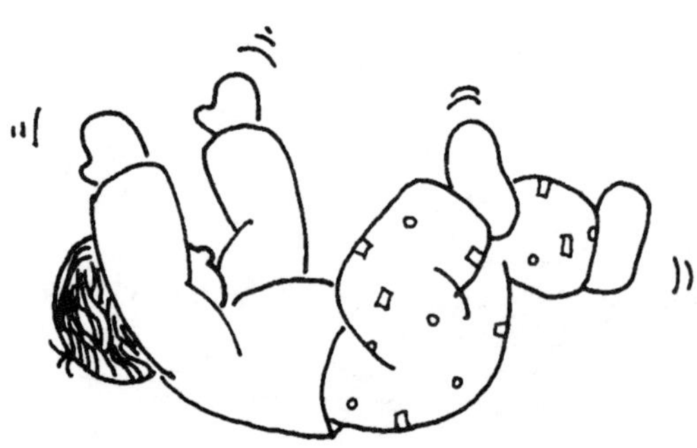

The Christmas Tree

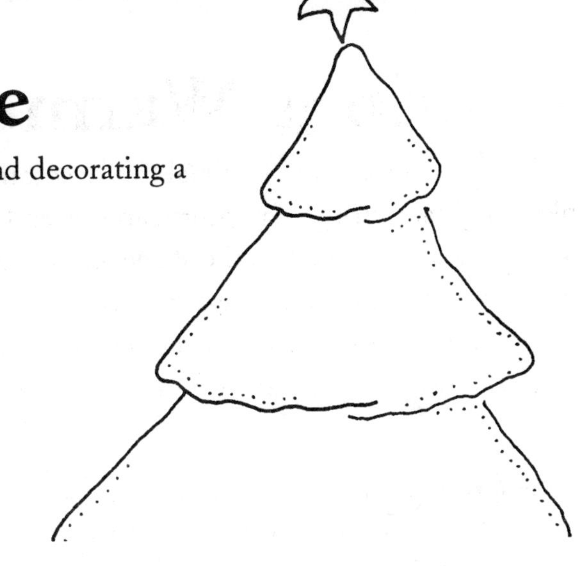

Have your children act out the motions of finding and decorating a Christmas tree while you read the following poem.

I went looking for a Christmas tree.
(Cup hand above eye and start walking.)

I went to find one that would please me.

The first tree I found was much too small.
(Bend down and measure small tree with hand.)

The second tree I found was much too tall.
(Raise hands up high.)

The third three I found was much too thick.
(Spread arms way out.)

The fourth tree I found was as thin as a stick.
(Hold up one finger.)

The fifth tree I found looked full and fine,
(Make the outline of a tree with hands.)

So I chopped it down and made it mine.
(Pretend to chop down tree.)

I took it home and set it up straight
(Pretend to set up tree.)

And then began to decorate.
(Pretend to hang ornaments.)

When I was finished, I could see

That I had picked the perfect tree!

Jean Warren

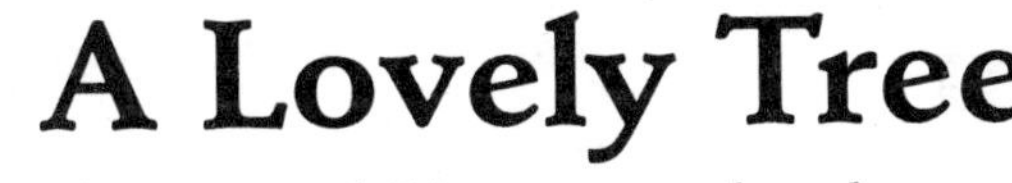

A Lovely Tree

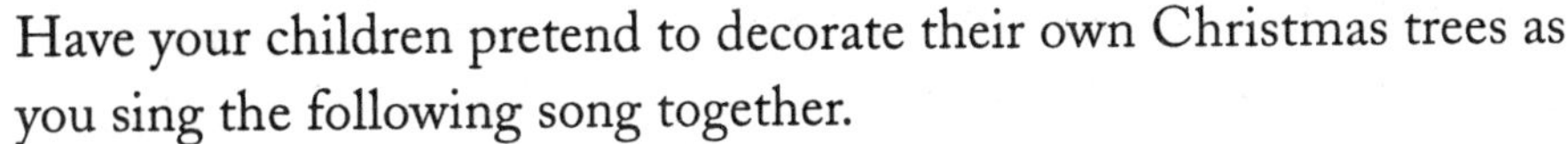

Have your children pretend to decorate their own Christmas trees as you sing the following song together.

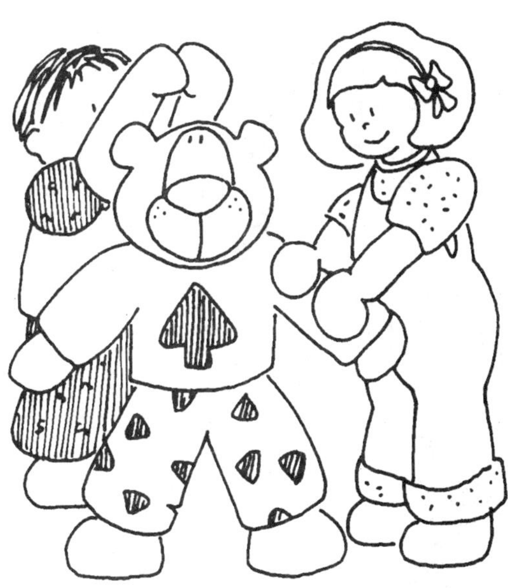

Sung to: "The Mulberry Bush"

Here stands a lovely Christmas tree,
Christmas tree, Christmas tree.
Here stands a lovely Christmas tree,
So early in the morning.

Here is a star for the Christmas tree,
Christmas tree, Christmas tree.
Here is a star for the Christmas tree,
So early in the morning.

Additional verses: Here are the lights for the Christmas tree; Here's tinsel to hang on the Christmas tree; Here's ornaments for the Christmas tree; Put presents under the Christmas tree.

Jean Warren

Running Warm-Ups

Your children's natural desire to run is channeled into a movement exercise in this activity. Discuss the many different ways people can run, such as fast, slow, forward, backward, in slow motion, in place, in a circle, on tiptoe, side by side with a friend, dashing in a race, with giant strides, with baby steps, like a deer, like a mouse, like a bear, like a monster, like a penguin, down or up a hill, in water or on snow, or on hot cement. Let your children pick their favorites to demonstrate for you.

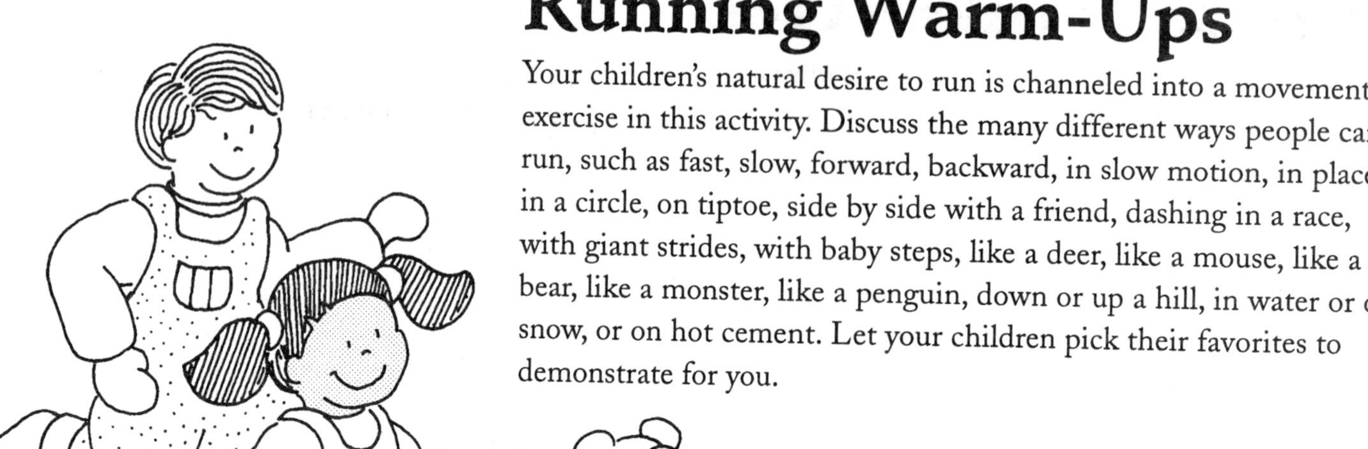

Santa's Team

Move from the running exercises above to this action story about how reindeer exercise to get ready to help Santa deliver all the toys at Christmas. Tell your children that each year before Christmas, Santa's reindeer have to get in shape for their long trip delivering toys. Only the fastest, strongest, and most agile reindeer will be able to make the difficult trip. The reindeer must practice many skills—running fast, darting quickly in and out of places, leaping across rooftops, and landing gently so as not to wake anyone.

Have your children pretend they are reindeer getting in shape for Christmas. (If you wish, make reindeer bells for each child by stringing several small bells on a piece of yarn and tying it to the child's wrist or ankle.) Do several calisthenics with the reindeer, including stretching and running in place. After your reindeer are warmed up, have them act out the motions to the poem on the following page.

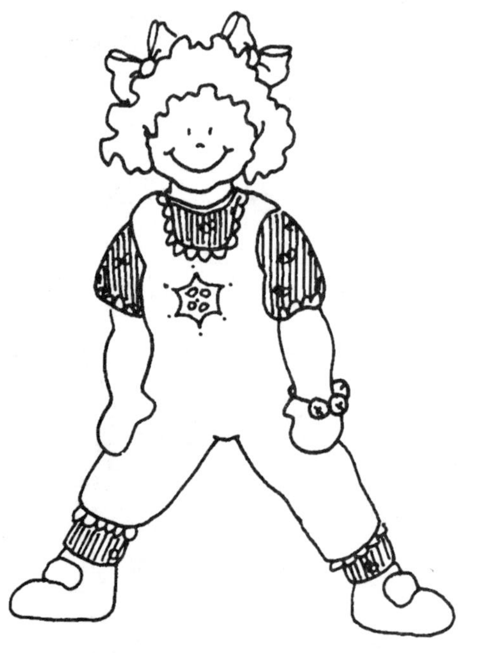

Reindeer Poem

Reindeer, reindeer, jump up high,
Reindeer, reindeer, fly 'cross the sky.

Reindeer, reindeer, softly on the roofs,
Reindeer, reindeer, lightly with your hooves.

Reindeer, reindeer, turn around,
Reindeer, reindeer, touch the ground.

Reindeer, reindeer, now run slow,
Reindeer, reindeer, still far to go.

Reindeer, reindeer, now run fast,
Reindeer, reindeer, home at last!

Jean Warren

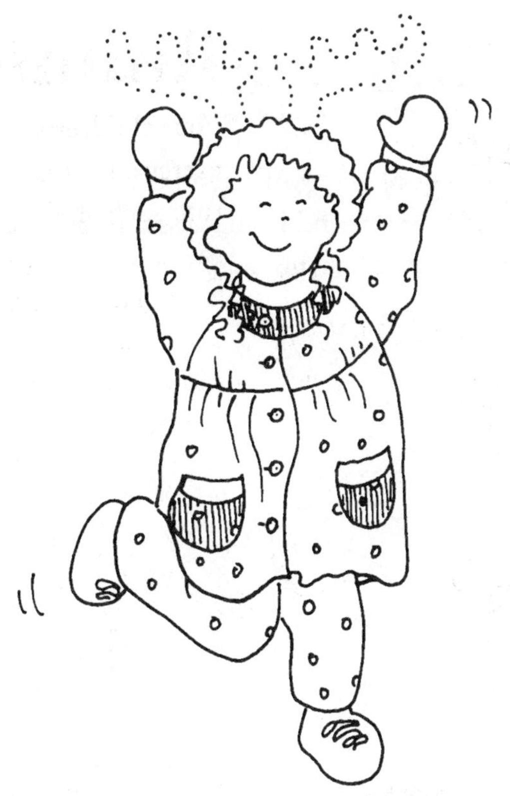

The Reindeer Dance

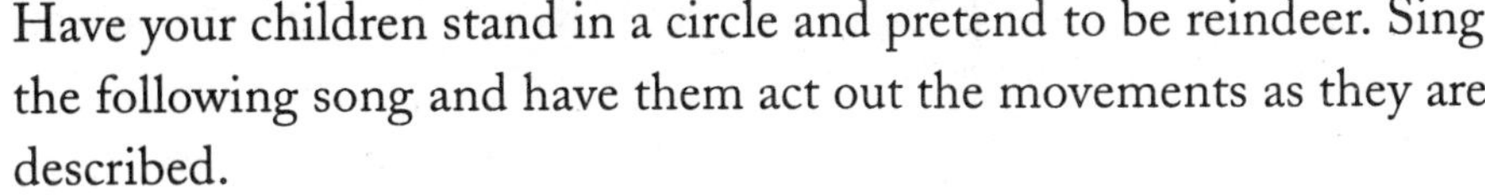

Have your children stand in a circle and pretend to be reindeer. Sing the following song and have them act out the movements as they are described.

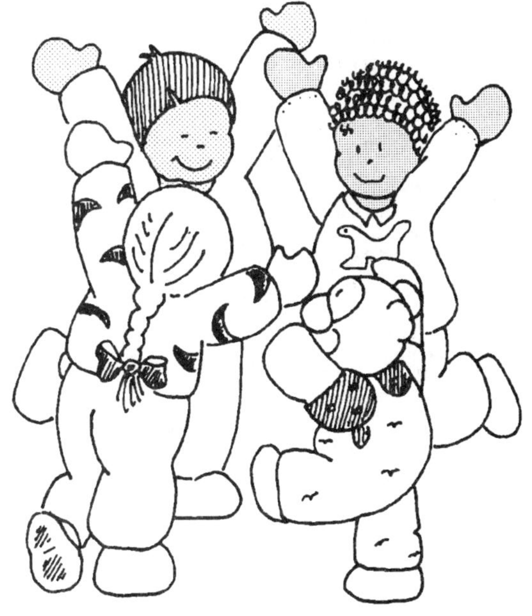

Sung to: "Hokey-Pokey"

You put your hooves in,
You take your hooves out.
You put your hooves in
And you shake them all about.
You do the Reindeer Dance
And you turn yourself around.
That's what it's all about.

Additional verses: You put your antlers in; You put your tail in.

Jean Warren

Snowball Warm-Up

Have your children lie on the floor and stretch out their arms and legs to form a blanket of "snow." Pretend to roll them up to make large snowballs. Have each child roll across the floor until he or she becomes very large and turns into a jolly snowman. Continue with the following activity.

Melt-Down Warm-Up

As you describe what happens, have your "snowman" children act out the motions. Tell them that when the weather is cold, snowmen are frozen and must stand straight and rigid all day and night. One day, however, the sun comes out, and it shines so long and so brightly that the snowmen begin to thaw. Have the children begin to "thaw," starting with their heads and working down to their toes as they slowly and gracefully melt to the floor.

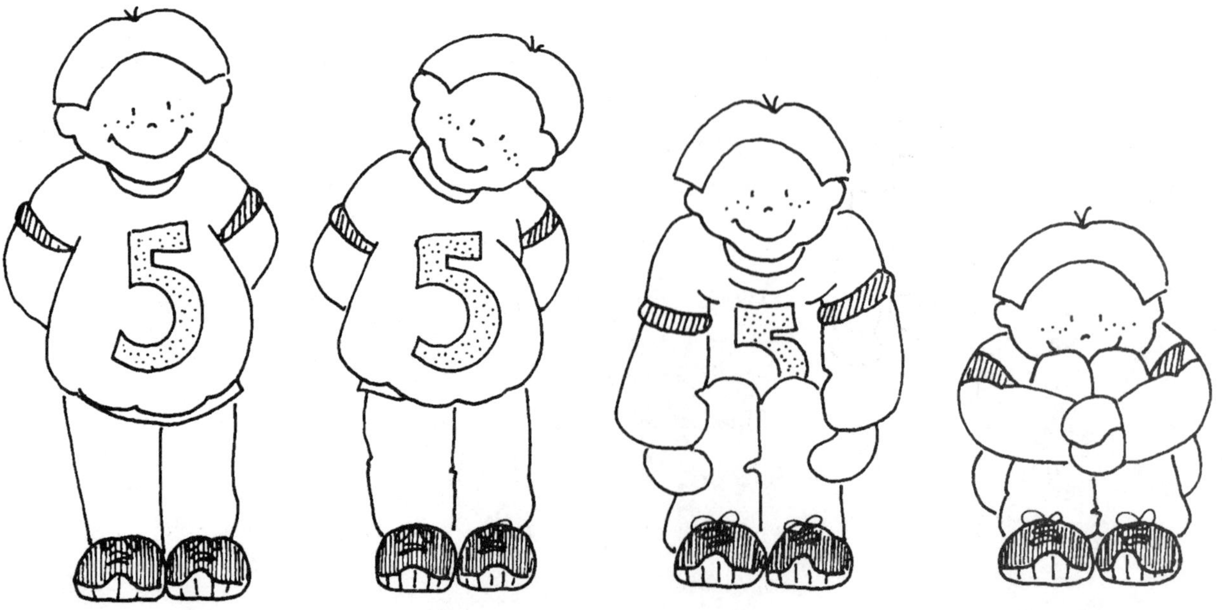

The Snowman

Sung to: "Row, Row, Row Your Boat"

The snow, snow, snowman
(Pretend to be a big, round snowman.)

Came out-of-doors to play,
(Pretend to open door and step outside.)

But the children cried, "Get back inside!

The sun is out today."
(Hold arms in circle above head.)

The snow, snow, snowman

Started to skip away,
(Skip in place.)

But as he skipped his body dripped
(Slowly lower body to ground.)

Until a puddle lay.
(Curl up body on floor.)

Jean Warren

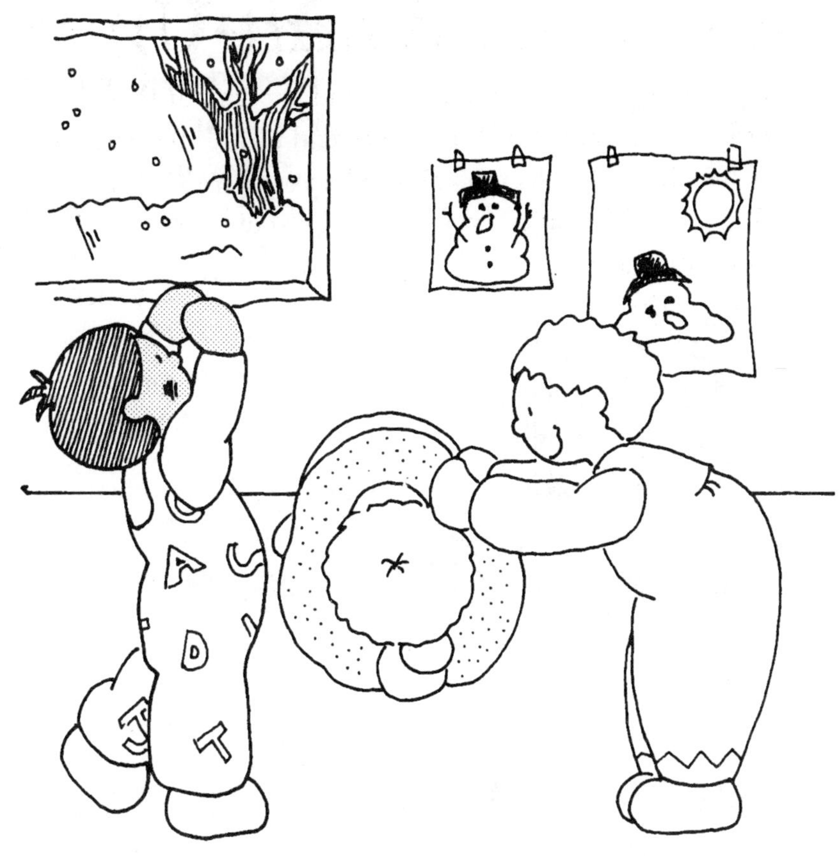

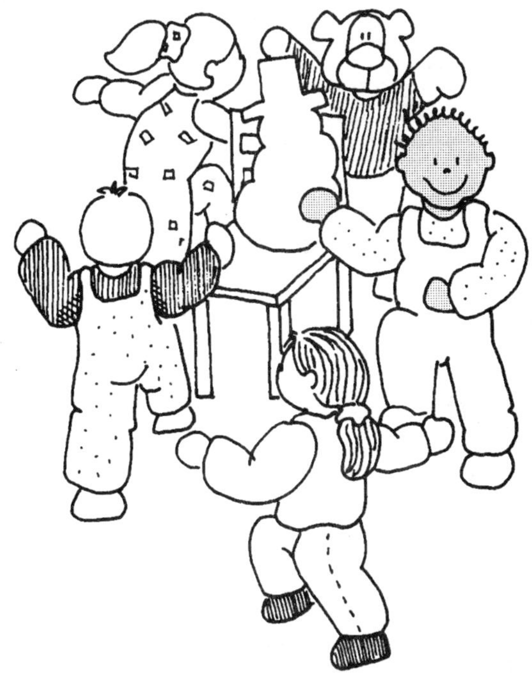

Dance Around the Snowman

Cut a large snowman shape out of white construction paper and tape it to a chair. Place the snowman chair in the middle of your room. Have your children stand in a circle around the snowman. Sing the following song. Encourage the children to move around the snowman in the manner indicated in the song.

Sung to: "The Mulberry Bush"

This is the way we dance around,

Dance around, dance around.

This is the way we dance around

Our snowman in the morning.

Additional verses: This is the way we skip; hop; sneak; spin; trot; crawl around.

Jean Warren

Sticky Warm-Up

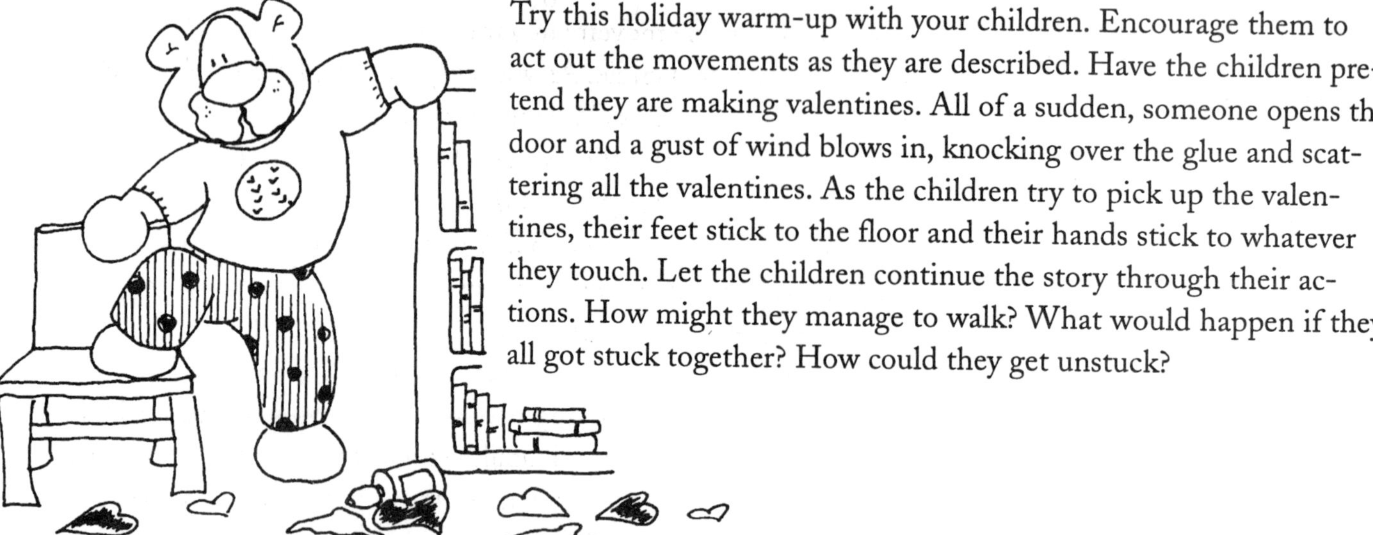

Try this holiday warm-up with your children. Encourage them to act out the movements as they are described. Have the children pretend they are making valentines. All of a sudden, someone opens the door and a gust of wind blows in, knocking over the glue and scattering all the valentines. As the children try to pick up the valentines, their feet stick to the floor and their hands stick to whatever they touch. Let the children continue the story through their actions. How might they manage to walk? What would happen if they all got stuck together? How could they get unstuck?

Delivering Valentines

Have your children pretend they are mail carriers delivering valentine cards and packages. How would they carry a huge box of candy? How would they deliver cards to someone who lives on top of a mountain? On an island? Underwater? In a tree house? On the moon?

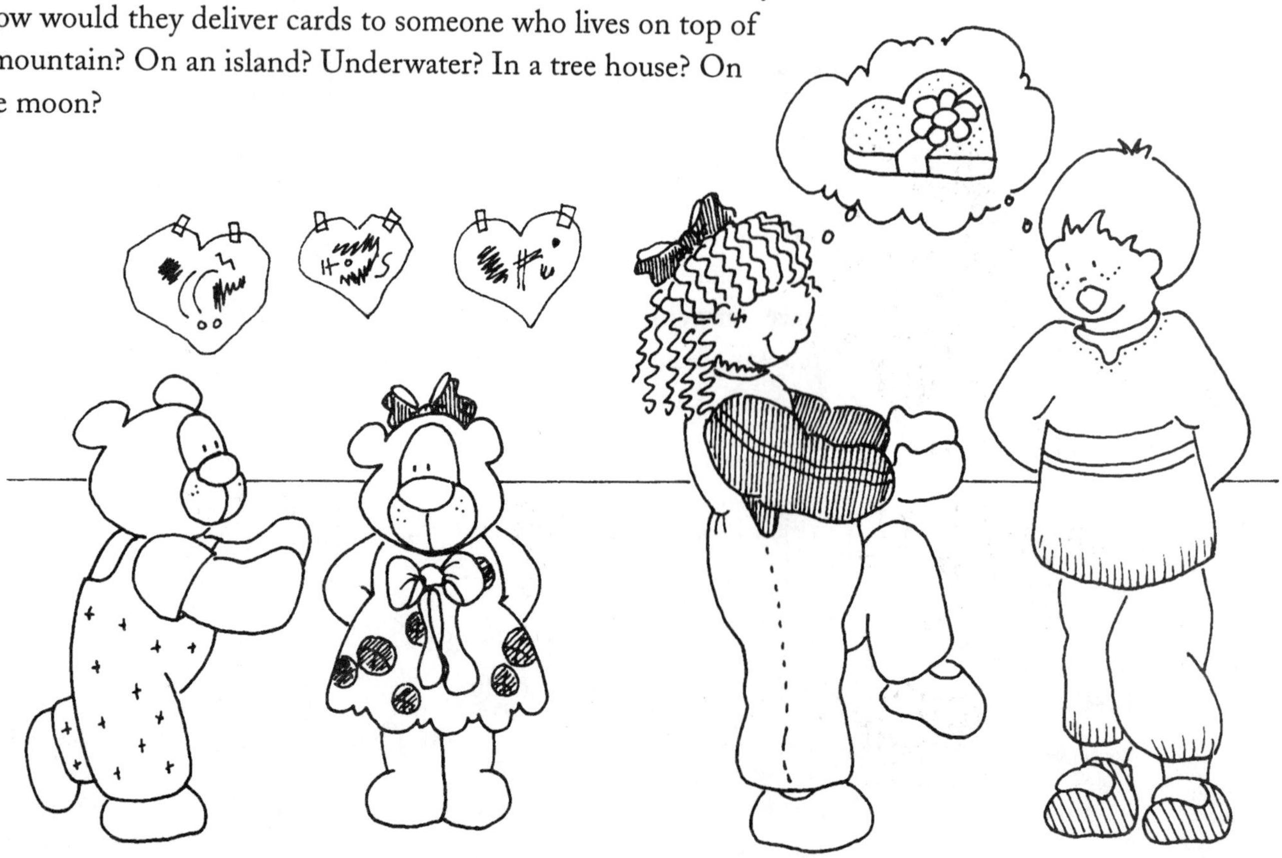

Here Is My Valentine

Play this valentine movement game with your children. Have the children stand in a circle. As you sing the song below, select one child to deliver a "sticky" valentine to his or her neighbor. Because the valentine is sticky, the two children stick together. Have the second child (who is still stuck to the first child) deliver another sticky valentine to his or her neighbor. Continue around the circle, until all the children are stuck together. Repeat the song as many times as needed. When everyone in the circle is finally stuck together, ask the children to think of ways they can get unstuck. For example, everyone can jump in a swimming pool and wash away the glue; everyone can pull away really hard; an adult can cut the valentines apart; or everyone can wait until the glue dries, then tear the cards apart.

Sung to: "The Mulberry Bush"

Here is my valentine,
My valentine, my valentine.
Here is my valentine
Just for you.

Here is my valentine,
My valentine, my valentine.
Here is my valentine—
I am stuck on you!

Jean Warren

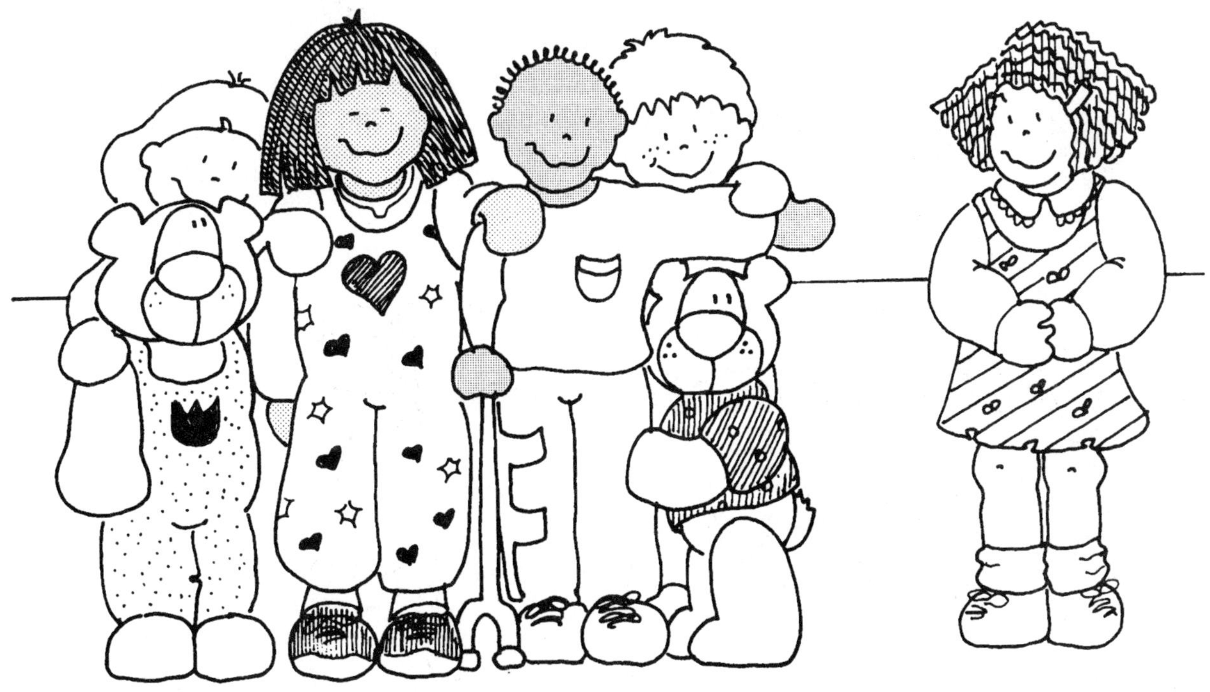

Shadow Warm-Up

Position a bright light to shine on you so that it casts your shadow on a wall. Show your children what a clever shadow you have—how it does everything you do. Show them how you can make your shadow wave, dance, twirl, and even fall down. Let the children take turns performing with their own shadows. If you wish, sing the following song as they perform, substituting the motion they are doing for *dance.*

Sung to: "Skip to My Lou"

Dance, dance, just like me.
Dance, dance, just like me.
Dance, dance, just like me,
Little shadow, just like me.

Jean Warren

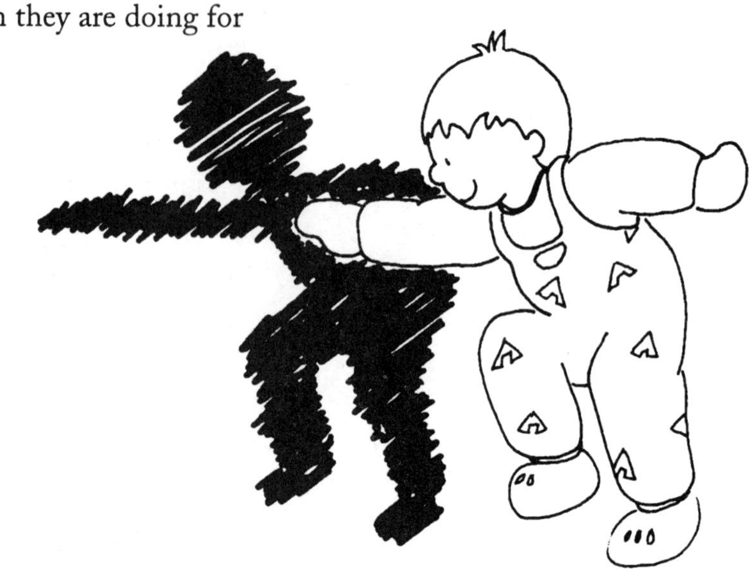

Shadow Partners

Extend the warm-up activity into a partner activity. Divide your children into pairs. Have the children in each pair face one another. Ask one child to move slowly while the other one, the shadow, tries to mimic what he or she is doing. After a few minutes, let the children switch roles.

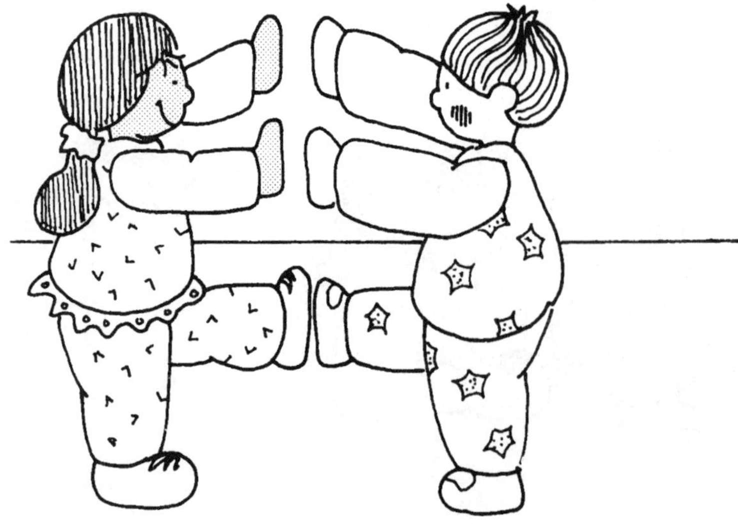

Little Shadow

Read the following rhyme to your children. Have them act out the motions as they are described.

There is a little shadow
That dances on my wall.
Sometimes it's big and scary,
Sometimes it's very small.
Sometimes it's, oh, so quiet
And doesn't move at all.
Then other times it chases me
Or bounces like a ball.

Jean Warren

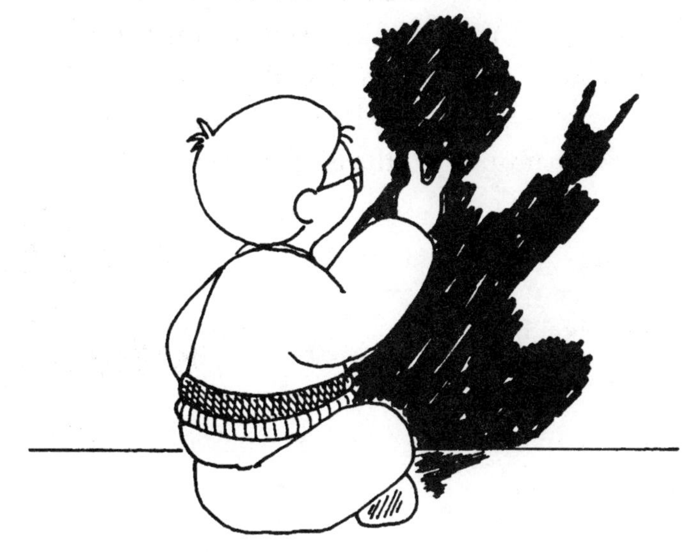

Groundhog Day

Tell your children the story of Groundhog Day. On February 2 every year, the groundhog wakes up from its long winter's nap and goes outside. If it sees its shadow, it is frightened and runs back inside its hole to sleep for another six weeks of winter. If it does not see its shadow, it stays outside to play, indicating that spring has arrived early.

Let your children take turns being the groundhog and popping up out of a hole (a large cardboard box) while you read the following poem. Let the child popping out of the box decide if he or she can stay or must run away.

Groundhog, groundhog popping up today.
Groundhog, groundhog, can you play?
If you see your shadow, run away!
If there is no shadow, you can play.
Groundhog, groundhog popping up today.
Groundhog, groundhog, can you play?

Jean Warren

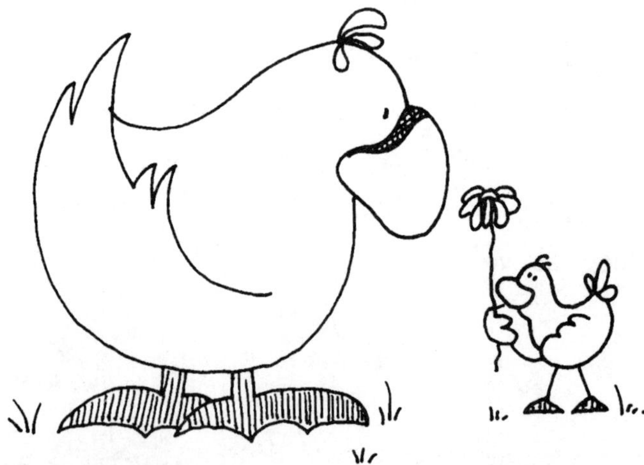

Spring

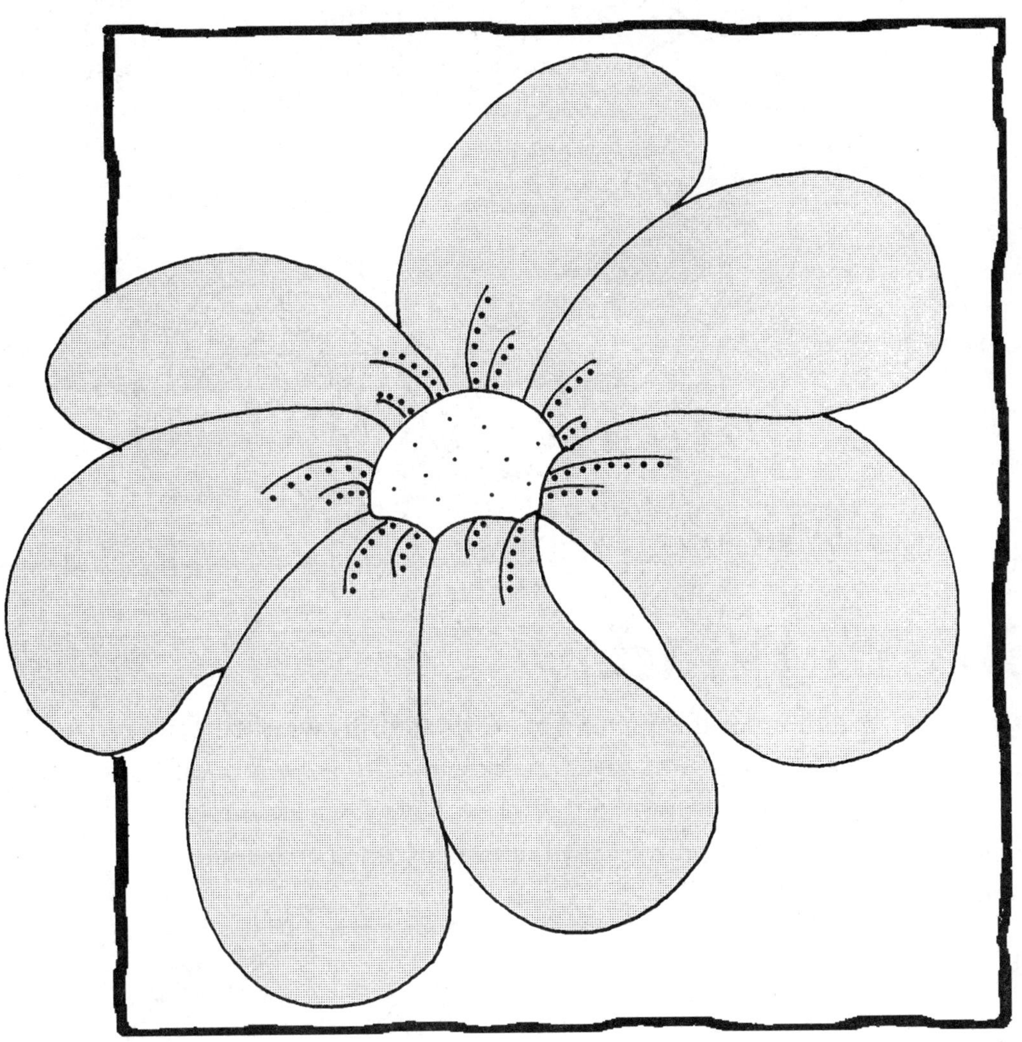

Scarf Warm-Up

Give each of your children a silk or nylon scarf. Ask: "What can your scarf do? Can you wrap it around yourself like a skirt and twirl? Can you make it disappear and reappear? Can you toss it up high? Can you run with your scarf over your shoulders? Can you make a flag blowing in the wind?" Then have the children pretend that their scarves are the wind. Ask them to show you how the wind can be a gentle breeze or a wild storm.

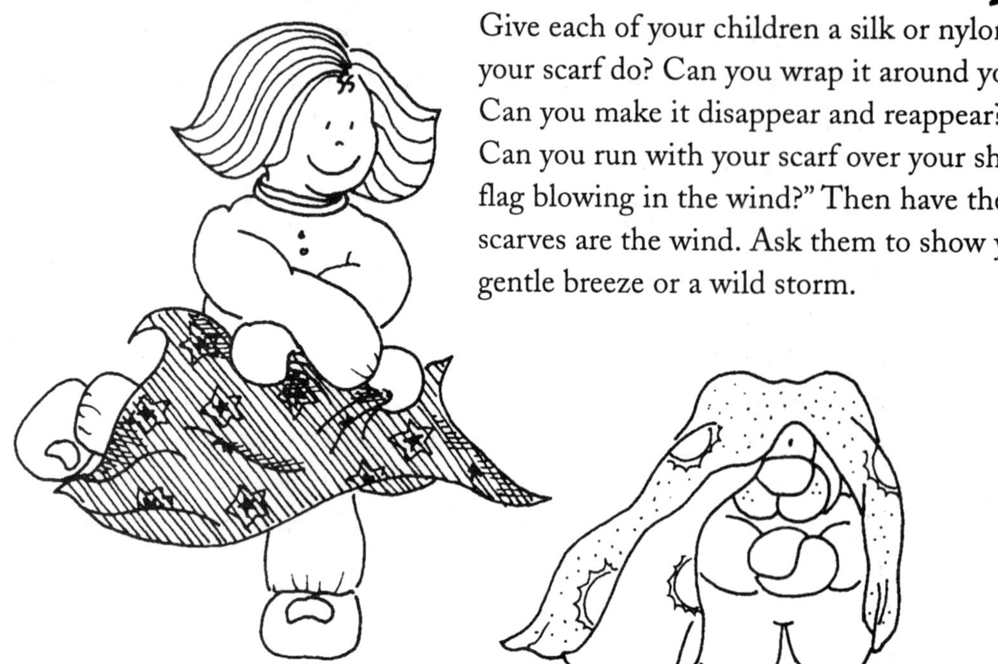

Storm Winds

Prepare your children for this pretend bout with stormy weather. Tell them that a hurricane has just arrived. Ask them all to move to a safe place in the room. As they move to that place, have them act out being tossed about in the wind, drenched with rains, and being spun around and around.

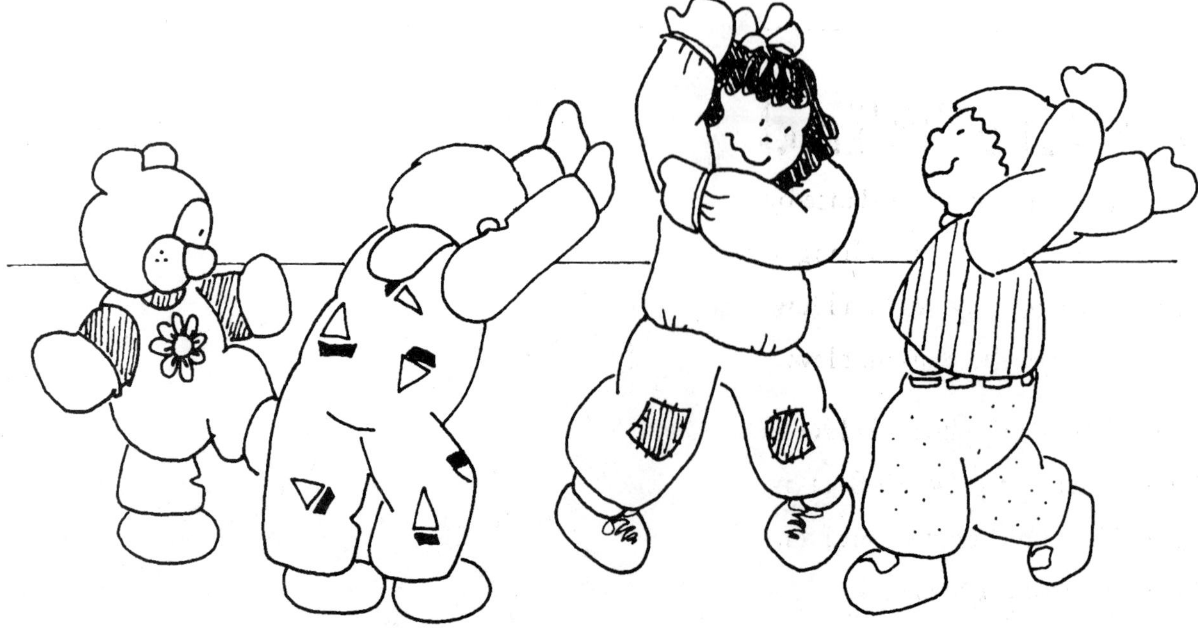

Clouds in the Breeze

Tie scarves or crepe-paper streamers to the arms of two children who will pretend to be the Wind. Have the other children pretend to be Clouds on a breezy day. As you describe the following scene, have the Wind and the Clouds act out their parts.

"Today is a beautiful day. The Wind is soft and gentle and the clouds are floating lazily around. Wait, the Wind is picking up now. There are little gusts here and there and the Clouds are bouncing up and down. Now the Wind is growing wilder and more fierce. The Clouds are scurrying across the sky, sometimes crashing into one another. (Be sure to set up some crashing rules ahead of time.) Gradually now, the Wind is slowing down and sending the Clouds lightly spinning. Finally, the Wind is completely stopped. The air is very still, and the Clouds are at rest."

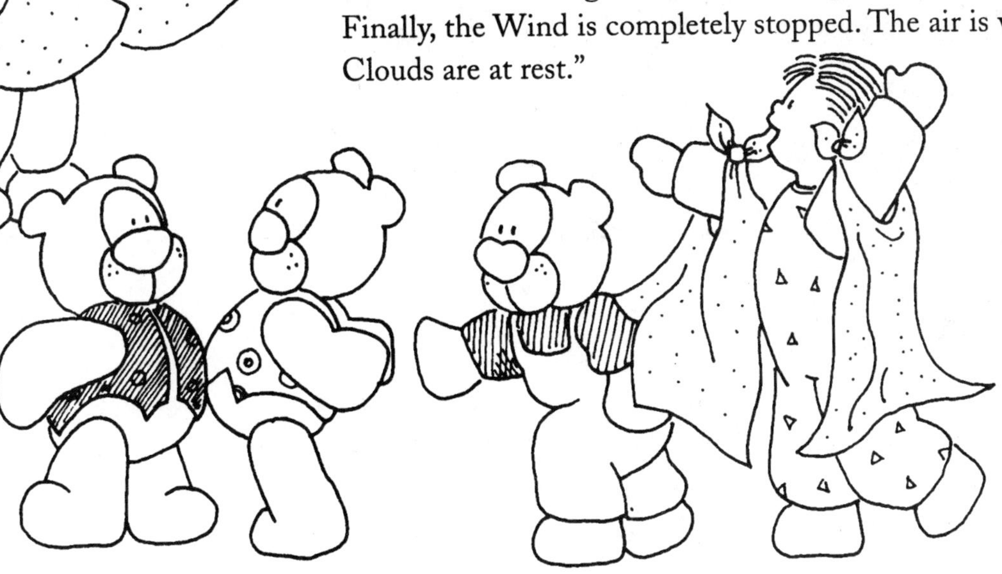

I See the Wind

I see the wind when the leaves dance by,
I see the wind when the clothes hang dry.
I see the wind when the trees bend low,
I see the wind when the flags all blow.

I see the wind when the kites fly high,
I see the wind when the clouds float by.
I see the wind when it blows your hair,
I see the wind most everywhere!

Jean Warren

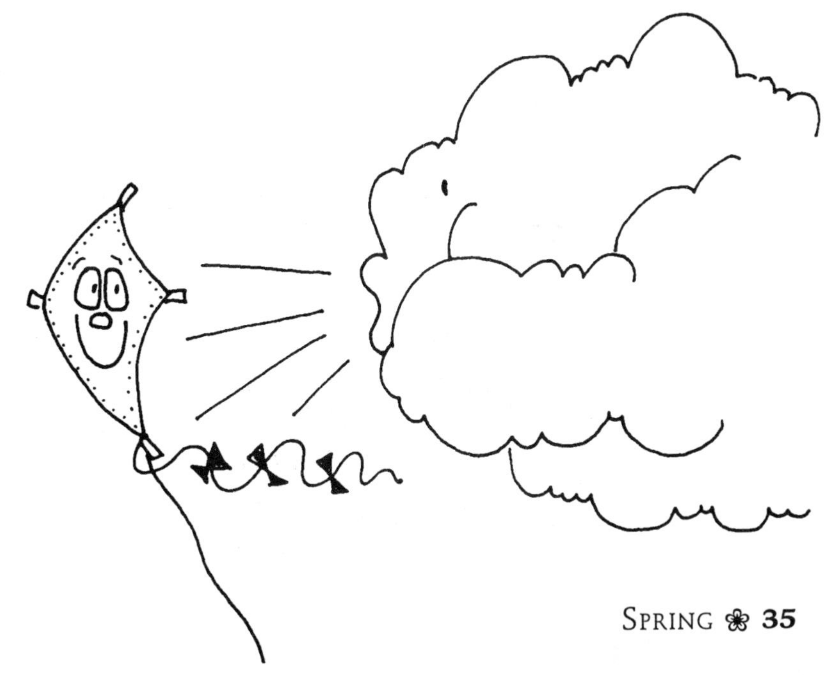

Reaching Warm-Up

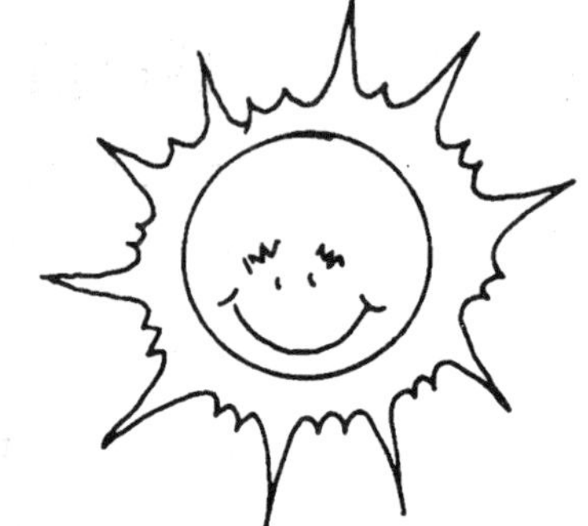

Ask your children to pretend to be little seeds, curled up tight in the ground. Slowly, have the children uncurl their bodies and stand up straight like seedlings. Tell them to imagine that the warm sun is shining overhead. Encourage them to reach, like seedlings, toward the light, stretching as high as they can. Now, ask the children to imagine that the sun is setting on one side of the room. Have them bend and stretch their bodies toward the light as it moves. Tell them that night has arrived and they can relax until the sun rises again and they stretch their bodies toward it.

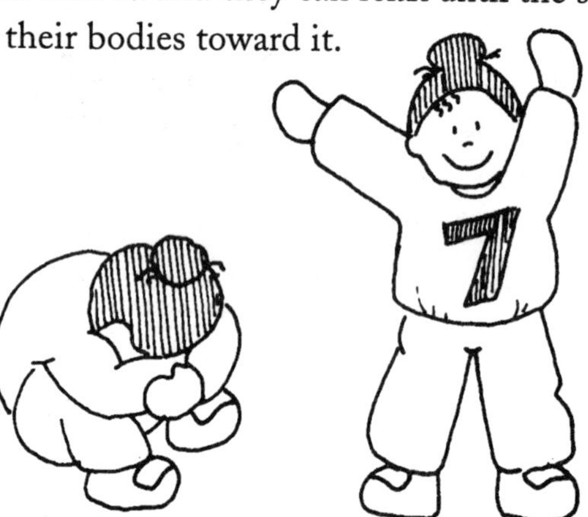

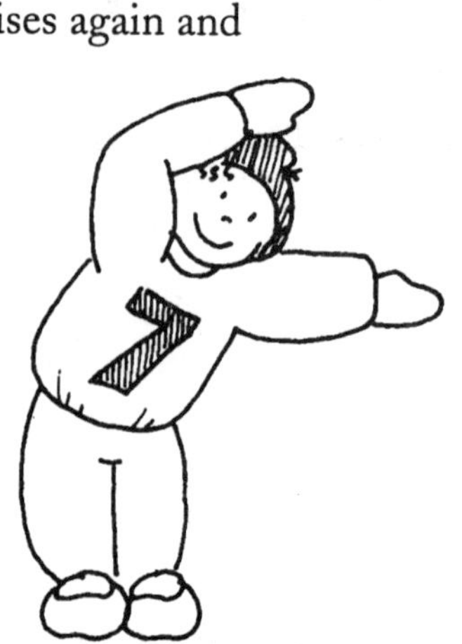

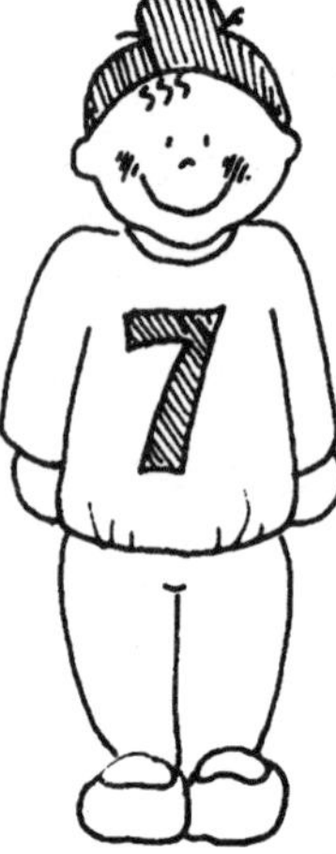

Flower Garden

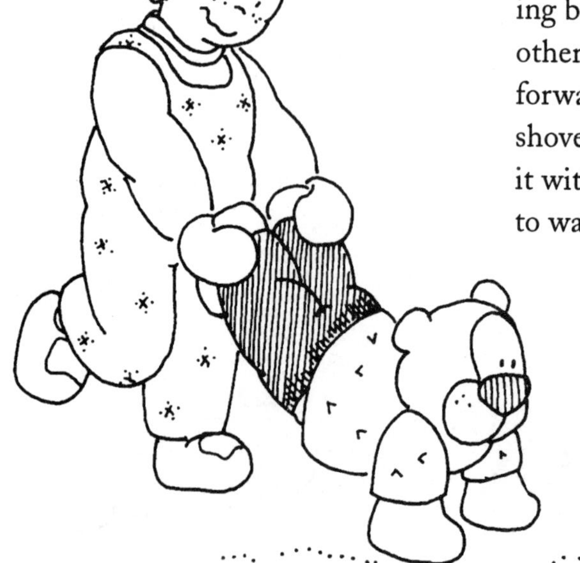

Have your children imagine that they are gardeners using an assortment of tools. First, have the children dig a flower bed with a shovel. Next, have them wheel over a load of fertilizer in "wheelbarrows." To make each wheelbarrow, have the children pair up, with one child lying belly-down on the floor and balancing on bent arms while the other child lifts the first child's legs and slowly propels him or her forward. After the fertilizer has been delivered, have the gardeners shovel it on the garden, work it into the soil with a hoe, and smooth it with a rake. Give them pretend seeds to plant and encourage them to water their gardens with a hose or a watering can.

My Garden

Let your children pretend to be the sun shining, the rain dripping, and the seeds growing as you sing the following song.

Sung to: "Skip to My Lou"

Sun in the sky, shine, shine, shine.

Sun in the sky, shine, shine, shine.

Sun in the sky, shine, shine, shine—

Help me make my garden.

Additional verses: Rain from the clouds, drip, drip, drip; Seeds in the dirt, grow, grow, grow.

Jean Warren

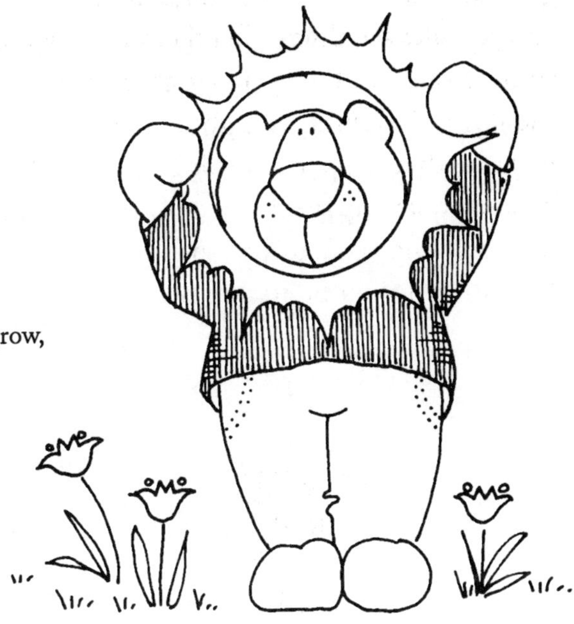

Flower Song

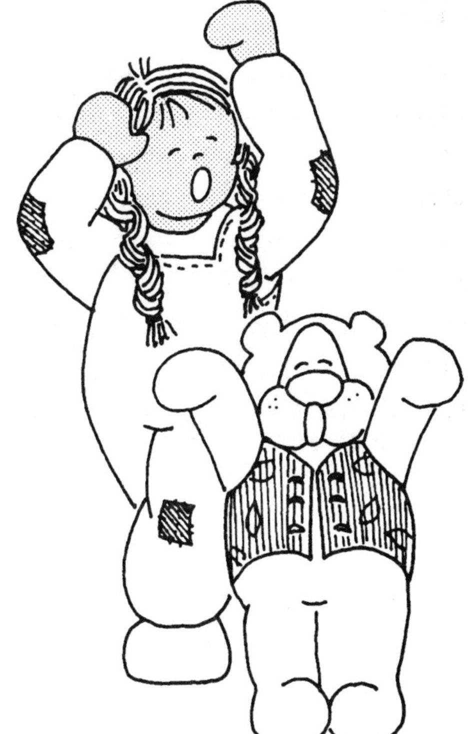

Sing the following song while your children pretend to be flowers and act out the motions.

Sung to: "The Mulberry Bush"

This is the way we wake up and yawn,

Wake up and yawn, wake up and yawn.

This is the way we wake up and yawn

When springtime is here.

Additional verses: This is the way we sprout our roots; pop through the dirt; stretch and grow; shoot up so tall; open our buds; bend in the breeze; smile at the sun.

Jean Warren

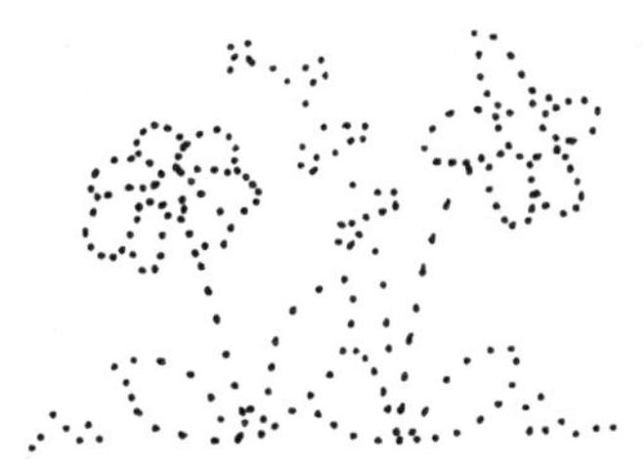

Hive Warm-Up

Ask your children to pretend that the room is a beehive and that they are all honeybees. As the queen or king bee, you will assign tasks to your worker bees. Make up beehive tasks that require large physical movements. For example, have some workers pour the nectar from flowers into pails, have others stir the nectar in a big pot to make honey, and have the rest sweep the hive. Before your busy bees have tired, appoint different children to take turns being the queen or king bee and to make up other imaginative jobs for the workers.

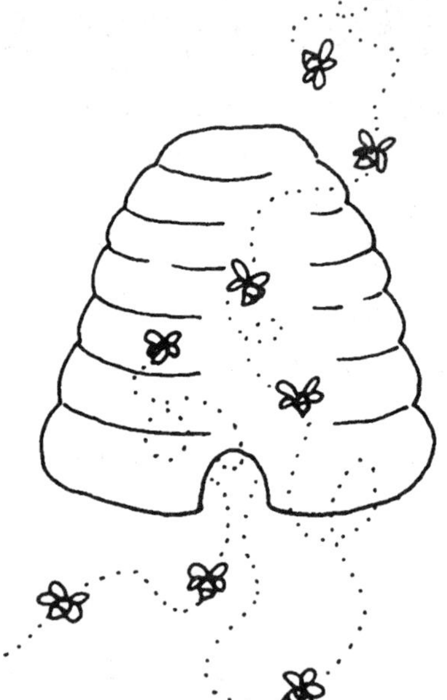

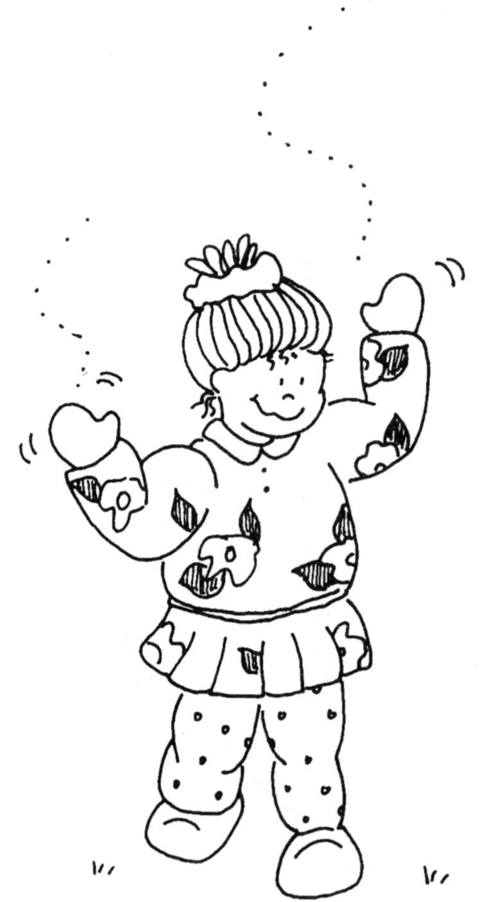

Dance of the Honeybee

Tell your children the following story. At the end of the story, let your children take turns being the honeybee and dancing directions to another patch of beautiful flowers.

"One day a honeybee was out looking for flowers when she happened to find a hidden valley full of the most beautiful blossoms she had ever seen. The bee hurried home to get her friends, but by the time she reached the hive, she was too tired to fly back to the valley. Instead, she did a special dance to show her friends how to find the flowers.

"The honeybee flew in one direction, flapping her wings ten times to show how many miles. Then she stopped and flew around in a circle once to show that at this spot there were a few flowers. Next, the bee flew off in a different direction, flapping her wings five times (for five miles). Finally, she stopped and circled many times to indicate that at this spot there were many flowers."

The Tiny Bee

Discuss with your children what it would be like to be very, very small. Let them pretend to be very little. Then, ask the children what it would be like to be very, very big. Let them all parade around as giants. Now read the following rhyme and let your children act it out. Let them expand on the rhyme if they wish, acting out other situations the bee may have encountered when she was big.

Once there was a tiny bee
Small and fuzzy and hard to see.

"Oh, woe is me," said the tiny bee.
"I wish I was huge, tall, and grand,
Bigger than all throughout the land."

And do you know what? Her wish came true.
She grew and grew and grew and grew.

"Oh, woe is me," said the giant bee.
"I cannot fly when I'm big as a tree!"

And the flowers all cried when she came to call,
For she squashed their petals and made them fall.

"Oh, woe is me, what shall I do?
I'll wish again, till my wish comes true."

And slowly, slowly, before her eyes,
She shrank back down to her regular size.

She soared up high and zoomed down low.
Now wherever she wanted, she could go.

The flowers all smiled as she flew by,
Happy to see their friend in the sky.

"Oh, golly gee, it's fun to be
Small and light and free as a bee!"

Jean Warren

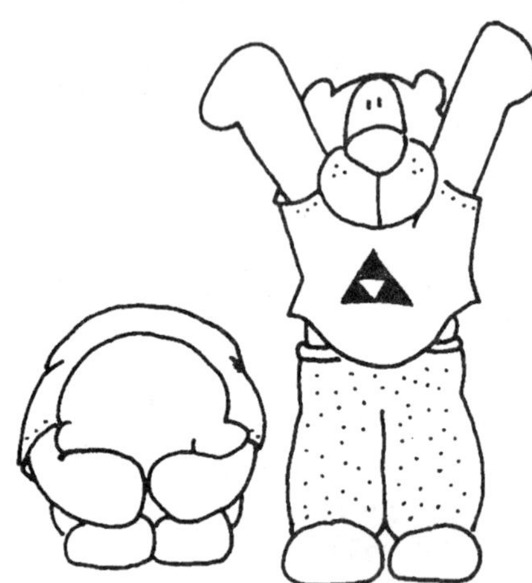

Jumping Warm-Up

Show your children a jack-in-the-box. Let the children pretend to be jumping jacks. Have them crouch way down in imaginary boxes. When you open up their "lids," have them jump out. Ask the children if they can think of any other ways a jack-in-the-box could jump out of its box. Let them demonstrate each of those ways for you.

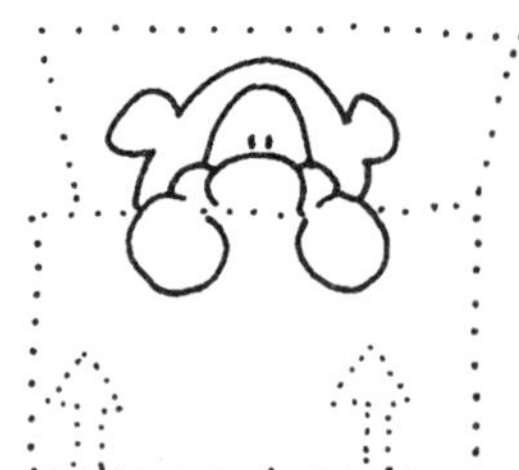

Animal Hop

Have your children pretend to be various kinds of jumping animals, such as kangaroos, bunnies, frogs, crickets, or fleas. Invite all of the jumping animals to an Animal Hop. Play some lively music as they jump all over the place. If you wish, show the children how to bend way down before they jump, spring up high, then land again in a crouch.

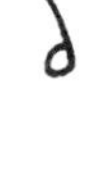

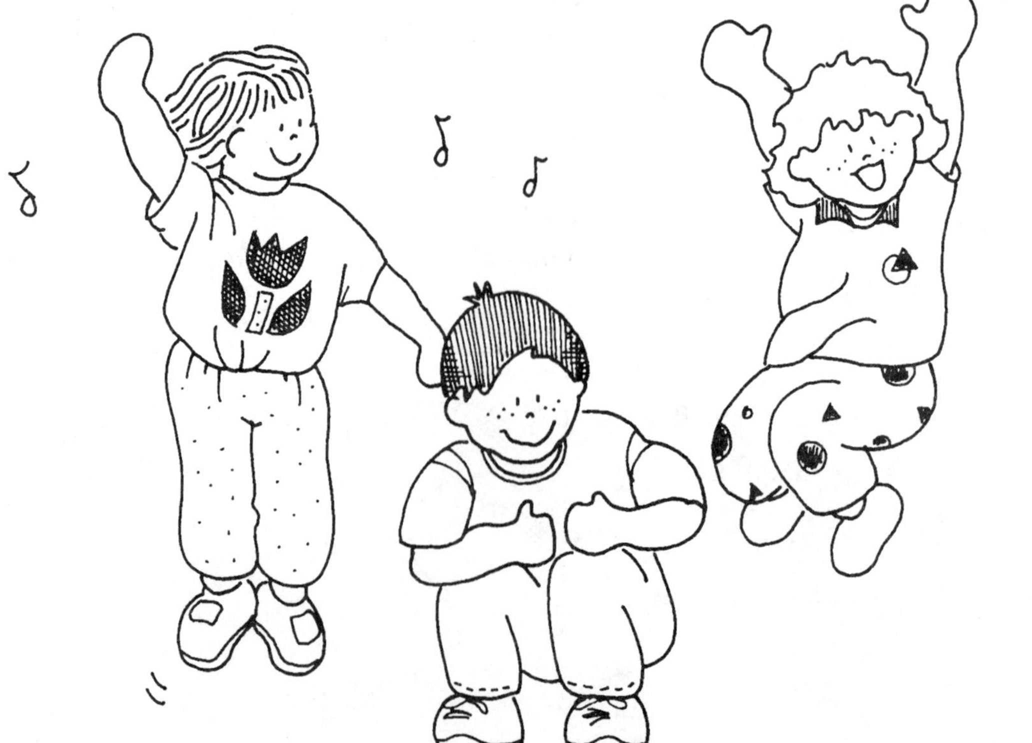

The Bunny Trail

Have your children pretend to be Easter bunnies. Tell them that they are in training now so they will be in shape to hop down the bunny trail and deliver baskets of eggs on Easter. Tell them they must practice these kinds of hopping: fast, slow, backward, high over tree stumps, low under fences, on one foot, and carefully while carrying a basketful of eggs. Next, show the children your bunny trail (it could be a masking tape line, a sidewalk, or a carpet-square path). Let each child decide how he or she would like to come down the trail. Sing the following song while the child moves down the trail, substituting the child's name and his or her movement for *jumping* and *Andrew.*

Sung to: "Mary Had a Little Lamb"

Jumping down the bunny trail,
Bunny trail, bunny trail,
Jumping down the bunny trail,
Here comes Andrew.

Adapted Traditional

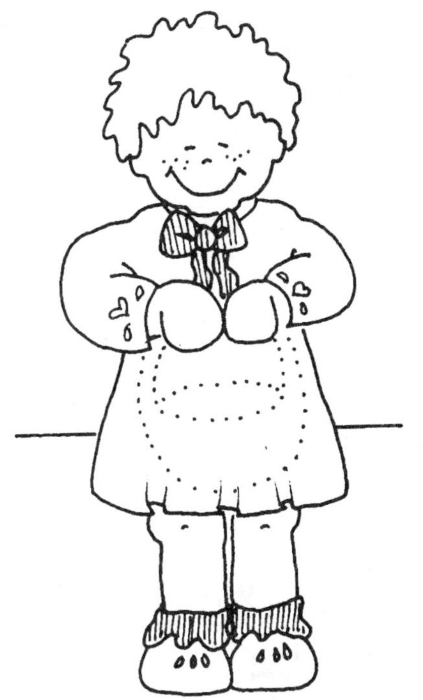

The Bunny Patch

Let your children pretend to pick up eggs and put them in baskets while you sing the following song.

Sung to: "The Paw-Paw Patch"

Hunt for Easter eggs and put 'em in my basket,
Hunt for Easter eggs and put 'em in my basket,
Hunt for Easter eggs and put 'em in my basket,
Way down yonder in the Bunny Patch.

Additional verses: Pick up colored eggs and put 'em in my basket; Pick up yellow eggs and put 'em in my basket; Pick up purple eggs and put 'em in my basket.

Jean Warren

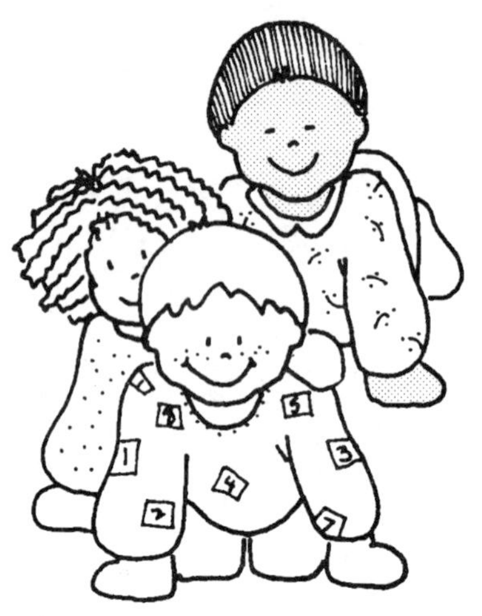

Caterpillar Warm-Up

Have your children get down in a crawling position and crawl in a line. Next, show them how to hook up by placing their hands on the back or legs of the child in front of them. Explain that each child is now a segment of one long caterpillar body. Have the children all start crawling with the same leg. See if they can crawl all around the room in this fashion. Some rhythmic music will help the crawlers co-ordinate their movements.

Grow, Caterpillar

Have your children pretend to be caterpillars and then butterflies as you sing and act out the following song together.

Sung to: "Row, Row, Row Your Boat"

Crawl, crawl, caterpillar,
You're such a fuzzy sight.
Don't you know, it's time to grow,
So crawl with all your might.

Spin, spin, caterpillar,
Spin a cocoon so tight.
Don't you know, it's time to grow,
So spin with all your might.

Wake, wake, caterpillar,
Break out into the light.
Don't you know, it's time to grow,
So break out with all your might.

Fly, fly, caterpillar,
It's time for your first flight.
Don't you know, it's time to grow,
So fly with all your might.

Jean Warren

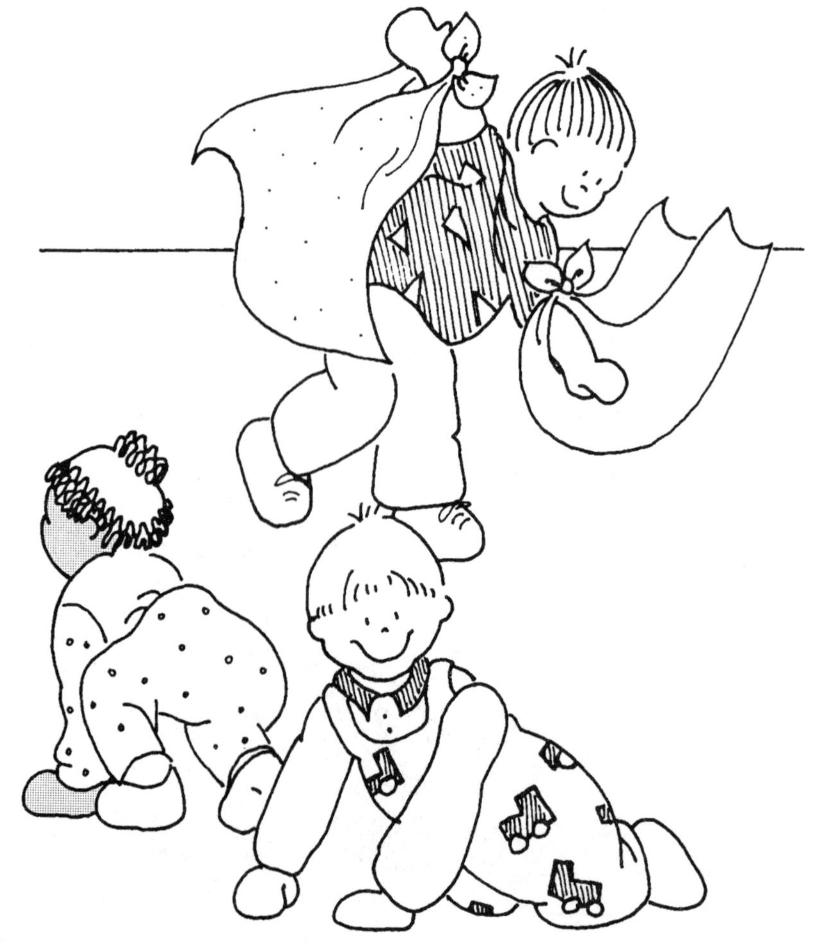

The Butterfly Story

Gradually lead your children into a dramatization of this butterfly story. Provide brightly colored scarves that the children can hide in their hands and unfurl as the butterfly emerges from its cocoon.

"One warm day, a caterpillar crawled up into a tree for a nap in one of the cool, green leaves. She curled up on the leaf and spun a web (or cocoon) around herself. In this cozy covering, she slept and slept.

"When the caterpillar woke up, she chewed her way out of her web. Suddenly she realized she no longer had her many legs. How would she ever get home?

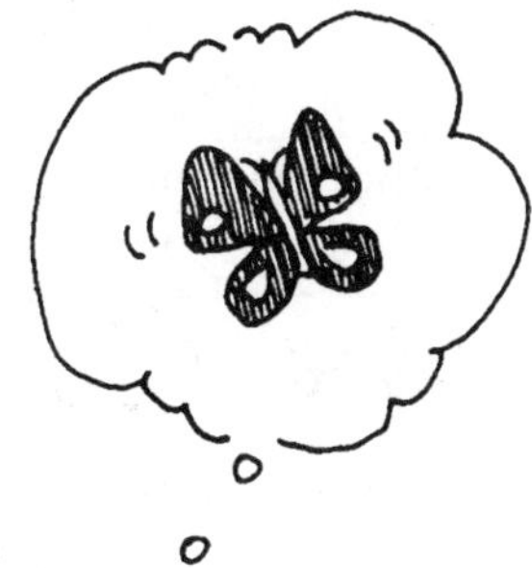

"The caterpillar started to cry. Then, as she tried to wipe her tears, she discovered to her joy that, while asleep, she had grown two beautiful butterfly wings. She opened her wings, flapped and flapped, and was soon soaring through the sky."

How does the story end? Where does the butterfly go and what happens to her? Ask the children to help you finish the story.

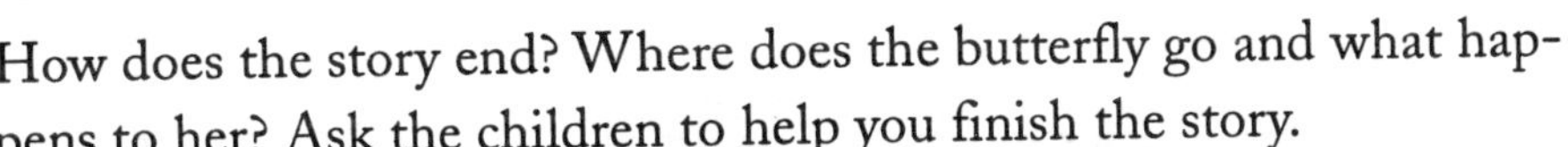

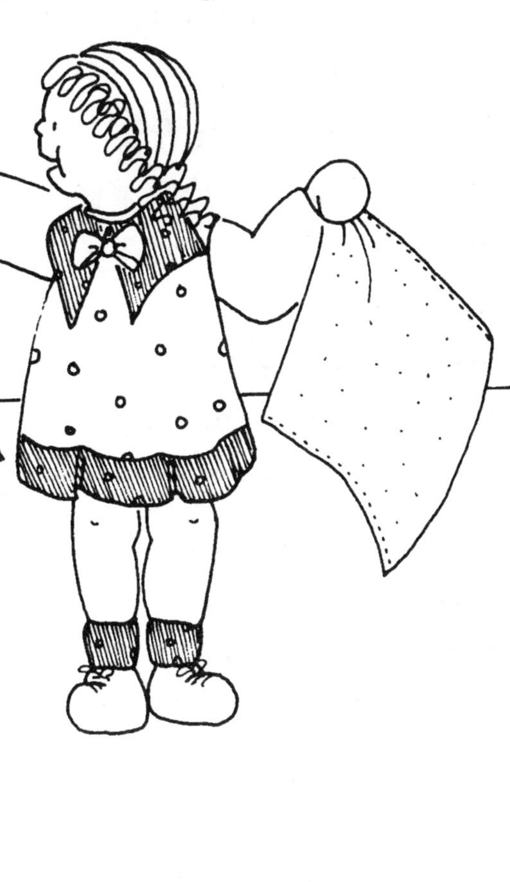

Wing Warm-Up

There is no prop that spurs children's imaginations more than a pair of wings. You can simply cut a pair of wing shapes out of construction paper and tape them to a child's wrists. Or safety-pin a long strip of fabric to a child's shirt at the neck and wrists. Make a set of wings for each child. Let your children experiment with their wings as you recite the following poem.

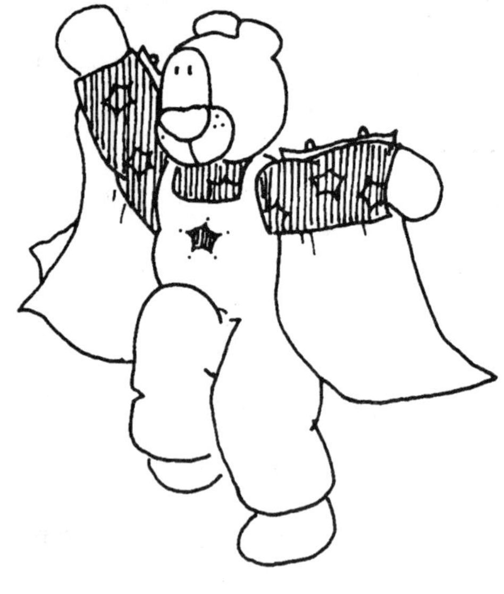

Flying fast, flying slow,

Soaring high, swooping low,

Swirling and twirling and gliding through the air,

The wings of a bird travel everywhere.

Author Unkown

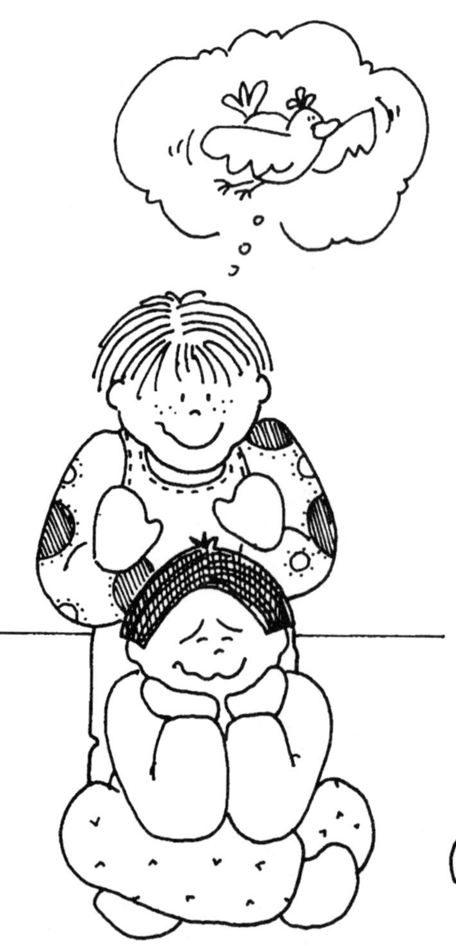

Learning to Fly

Tell your children the following story.

"A mother bird has been sitting on her nest of eggs. One day the eggs hatch, and the mother bird busies herself with finding food and feeding her babies. At last she decides they are big enough to learn to fly. She flies around the nest and shows her babies how it is done. Soon all the little birds are flying but one, who is afraid. How can the mother bird get her baby to fly?"

Have your children come up with possible solutions to help the baby bird learn to fly. For example: push the baby out of the nest, send up a sneaky cat to scare the baby into flying away, or have two other birds hold onto the baby's wings to help it fly. Encourage the children to retell the story with the agreed-upon ending, acting out as many elements of the story as they can (pecking their way out of an egg, flapping their baby wings, and so on).

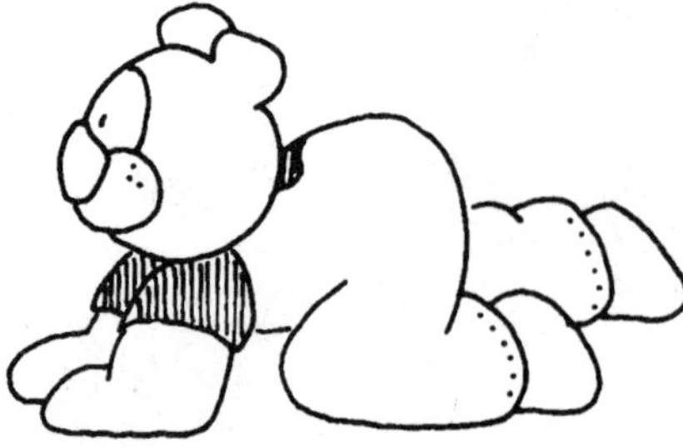

Four Little Birds

Four little birdies high in the tree,
One flew away, then there were three.

Three little birdies with feathers so new,
One flew away, then there were two.

Two little birdies out in the sun,
One flew away, then there was one.

One little birdie alone in the nest,
Afraid to fly out and join the rest.

Come little birdie, come fly like me,
Come little birdie, fly out of the tree.

Flap your wings up, flap your wings down
So you can fly over field and town.

Up, up, and away the birdie did fly,
Up over the trees, up into the sky.

Four little birdies now up so high
I almost forgot to wave them "goodbye!"

Jean Warren

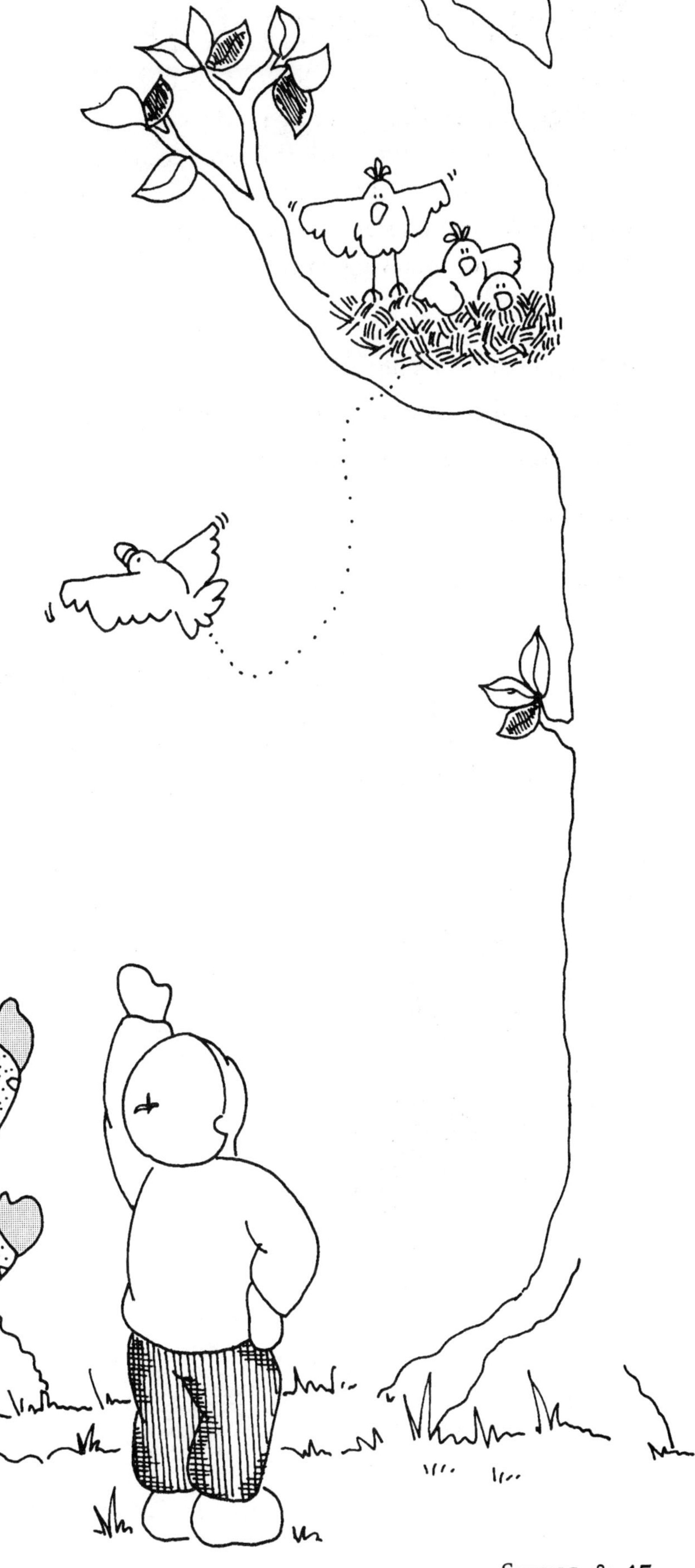

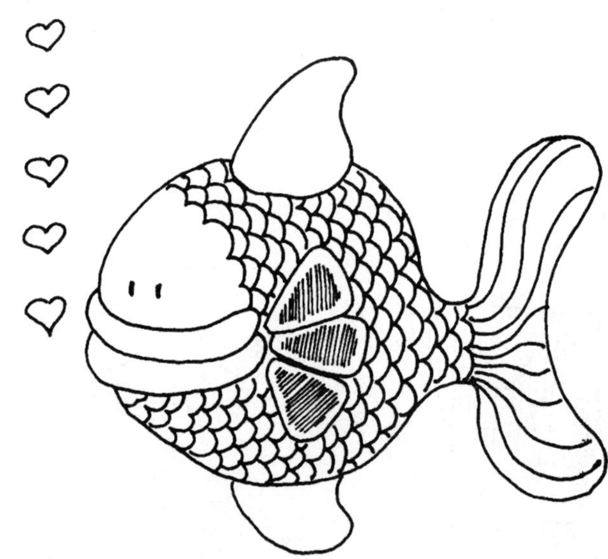

Summer

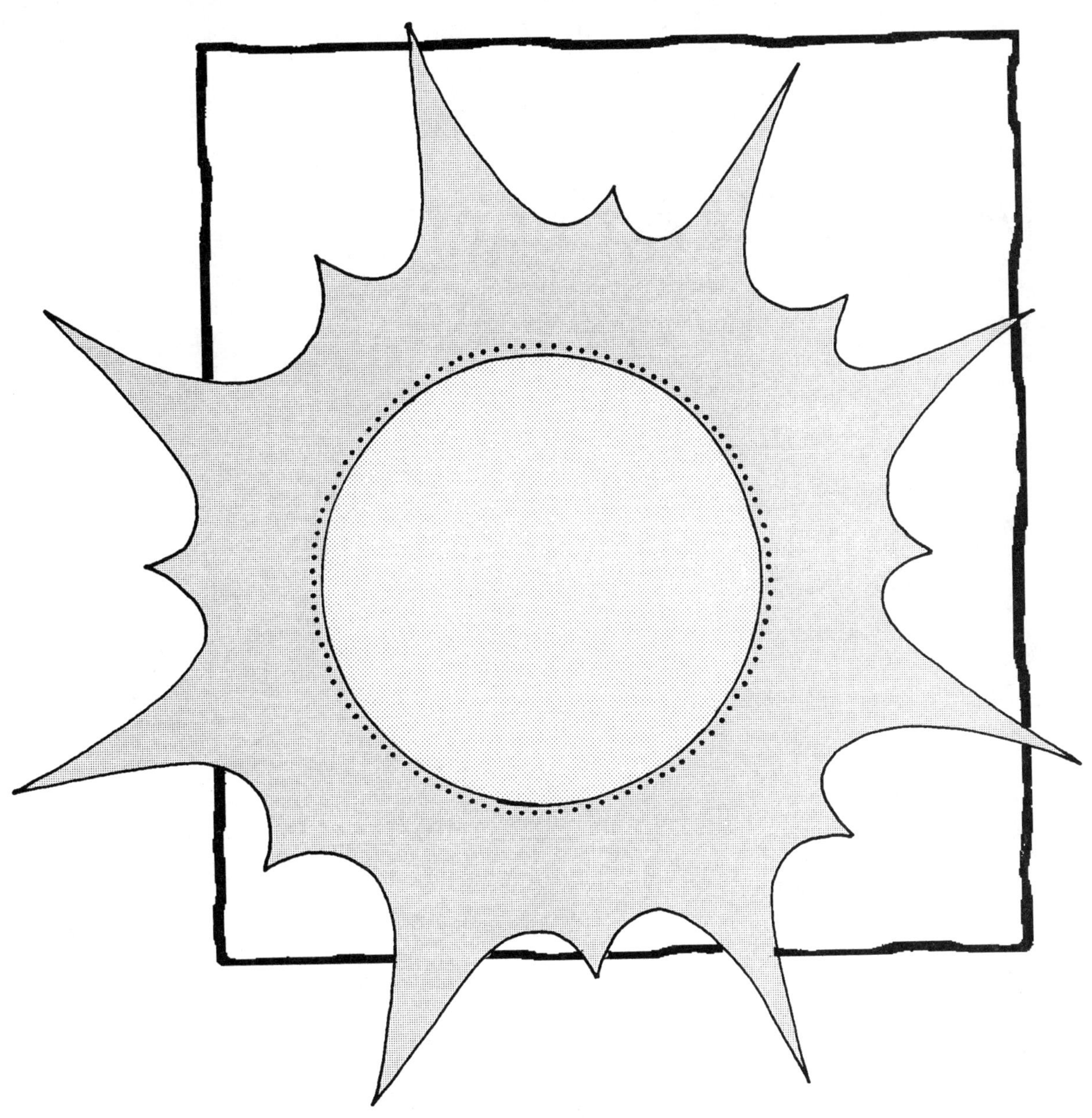

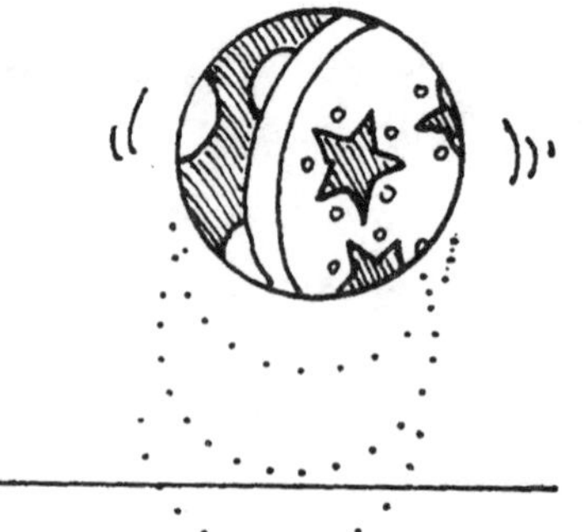

Bouncing Warm-Up

Have your children pretend that they have accidentally swallowed a bouncing rubber ball. Encourage them to dramatize what might happen as the ball moves inside their bodies. How would their shoulders bounce? Their elbows? What would happen if the ball was in one of their feet? You may wish to play some music as the children bounce along.

At the Playground

Sing the following song while your children are at a real playground, or have them act out the different motions that are described.

Sung to: "Row, Row, Row Your Boat"

Pump, pump, pump the swing,
Pump as high as you can.
You pump so high
You touch the sky—
Then down you come again.

Climb, climb, climb the bars,
As many as you can.
You climb to the top,
And then you stop—
Then down you climb again.

Ride, ride, ride your trike,
Ride as fast as you can
All the way round
The whole playground—
Then round you go again.

Jean Warren

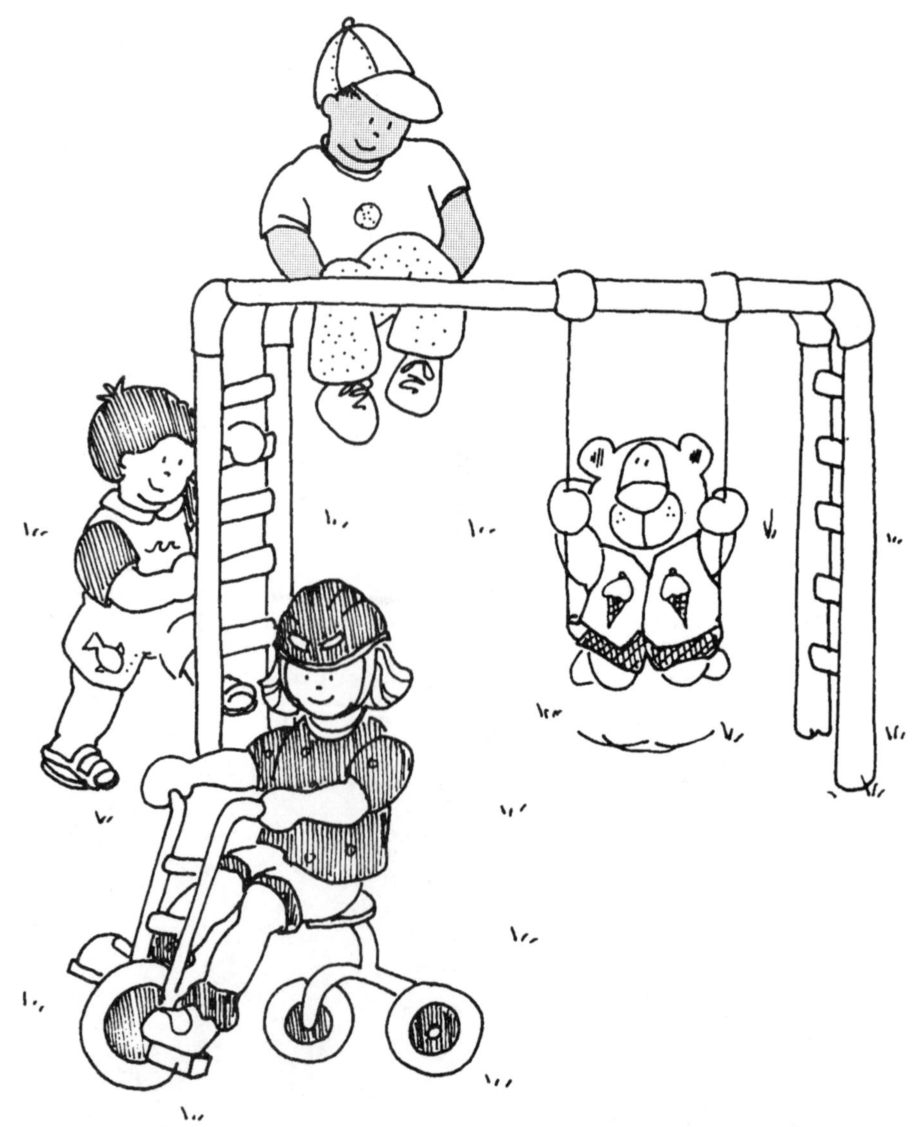

Playground Equipment

Invite your children to help build an imaginary playground. Ask them to name some equipment they would like to have. Next, help the children figure out ways to use their bodies to make the equipment. Below are some examples.

- Have the children make swings by holding their arms at their sides and swinging them back and forth. Or have two children face each other and hold hands to form a swing for a teddy bear or a doll.
- Line up several children, then have them bend over and put their hands on the ground to form a tunnel. Let the other children crawl through it.
- Have the children hold their arms straight out to the sides and move them up and down like a seesaw.
- Ask the children to sit on the floor with their legs bent to make a slide. Let them take turns sliding a teddy bear or a doll down their legs.
- Let the children form basketball hoops with their arms. If you wish, give the children soft foam balls to toss into one another's "baskets."

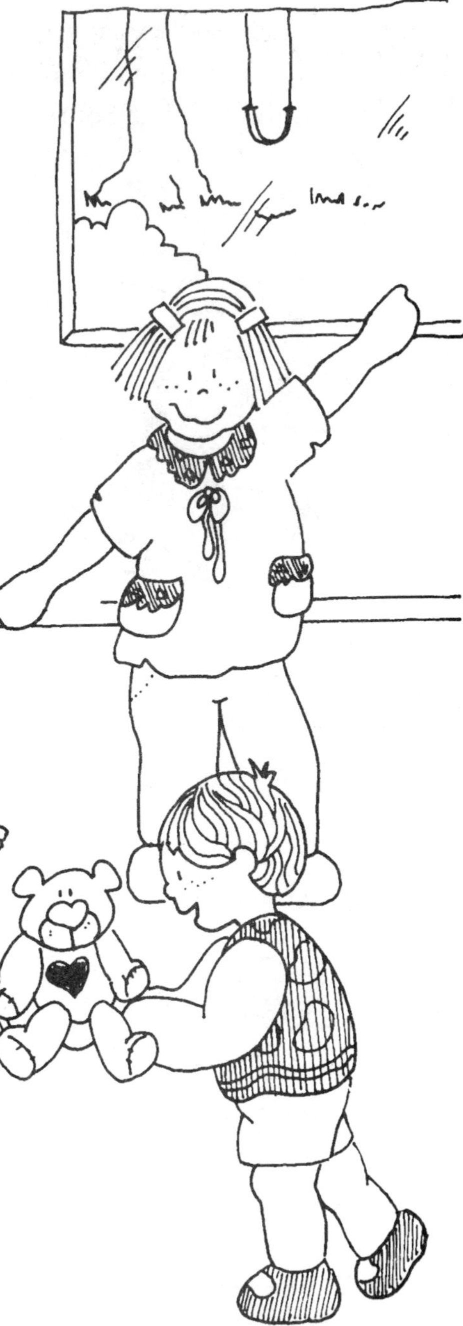

Water Warm-Up

Help your children get in the mood for some water fun. First, ask them to show you as many different ways to swim as they can think of. Next, have them imagine they are playing in water that is up to their ankles. How would they move around? How would they move in water up to their waist? Up to their neck?

Now, pass out pretend water masks and have your children slip them on and dive under water. What do they see? As they stroke through the water with their arms, have the children take turns naming something that they might see, such as fish, plants, sharks, or shells. If you wish, ask half of the children to be tall, willowy plants under the water and the other half of the children to swim carefully between them.

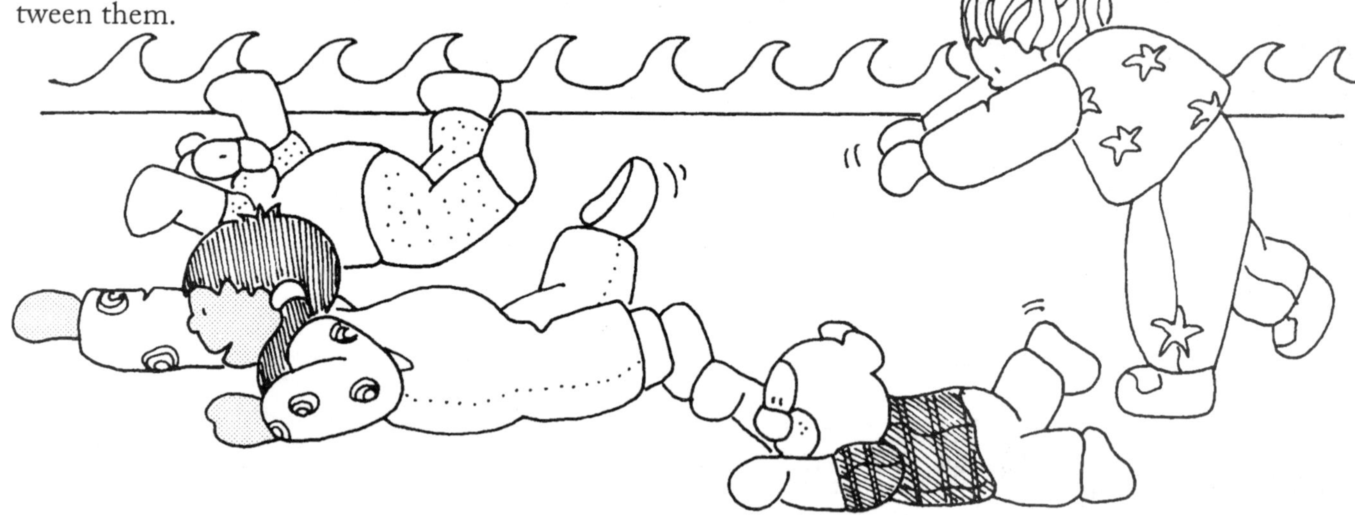

Swimming Song

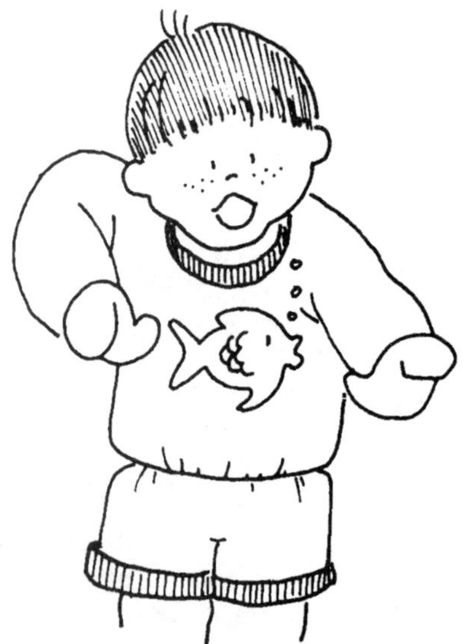

Encourage your children to act out the motions as you sing this swimming song to them.

Sung to: "Sailing, Sailing"

Swimming, swimming over the ocean blue,
I love to dive, I love to kick.
How about you?
Sidestroke, back float—underwater, too.
Swimming is so much fun.
It's what I love to do!

Jean Warren

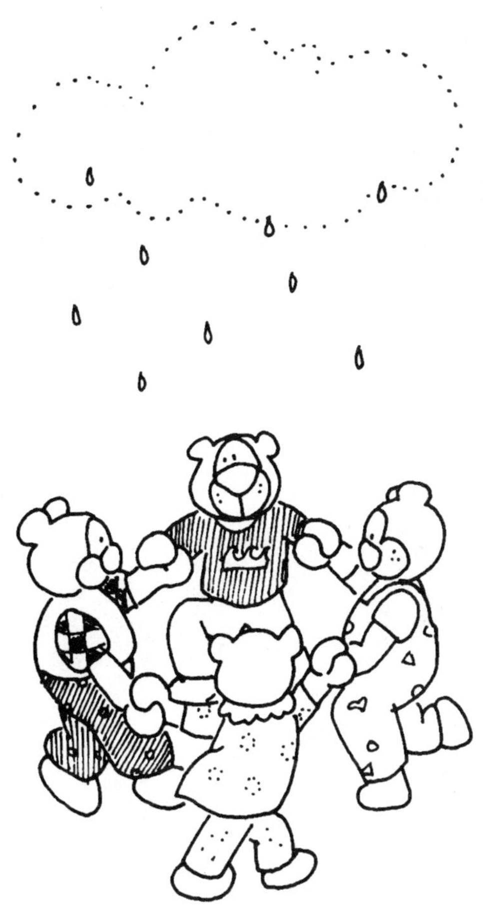

Water Cycle

Tell your children that they are going to help you act out what happens to a raindrop after it has fallen to the ground. Ask your children to imagine that they are those raindrops. Have them circle slowly around the room, joining hands with other raindrops next to them to form several small streams. Ask the streams to continue circling, each connecting with another stream to form a few rivers. Have the rivers move faster and faster, pretending to cascade over large rocks. As the children move with more speed and bumpier motions, have them move their heads, arms, and knees up and down to show the current.

As the rivers pass a designated spot, have the children turn into whirlpools, forming small four-person circles and twirling about. Eventually, have all the children hold hands and flow into the ocean, forming one large circle. Have the children slowly come together with arms raised, then flow backward with graceful arm movements to represent the tides.

As the sun shines over the ocean, have the children once again become drops of water that rise back up into the sky to form rain clouds.

Crossing a River

Encourage your children to think of some of the ways there are to cross a river, and then let them act out a few of them. For instance, they could step on stones or walk on logs to cross the river, jump over it, row a boat or paddle a canoe across it, or swim across it. You may wish to make a "river" in your room by putting two strips of masking tape on the floor several feet apart.

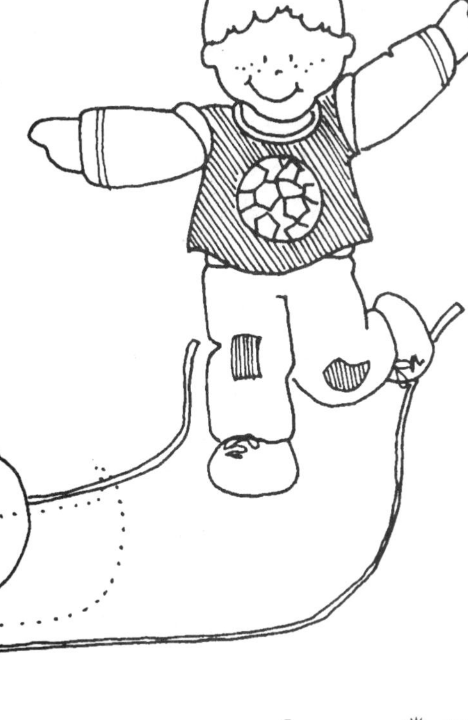

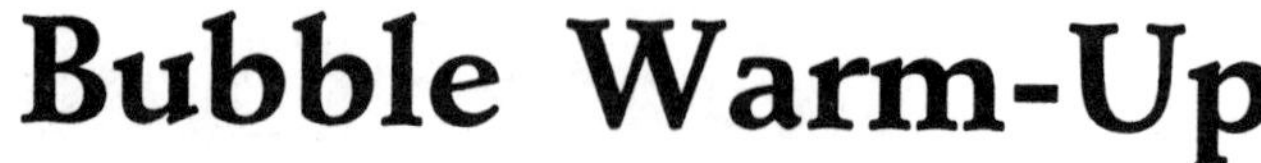

Bubble Warm-Up

Have your children sit quietly while you blow some bubbles. Ask them to observe what the bubbles are like and how they move. Now bring out a large Hula-Hoop. Tell the children that this is your giant bubble wand. As you slowly wave the wand, have the children move through the hoop, emerging as beautiful bubbles. Let the children float around the room awhile, eventually settling down to the ground with a gentle pop.

Magic Bubble Rides

Have each of your children pretend to crawl inside a magic bubble that can take them wherever they want to go. Perhaps they will want to roll and bob about over the ocean, fizz with the other bubbles in a bottle of soda, sit on the back of an elephant for a ride through the jungle, or perch on the wing of an airplane as it soars through the sky. Encourage the children to act out different situations where their bubbles might take them.

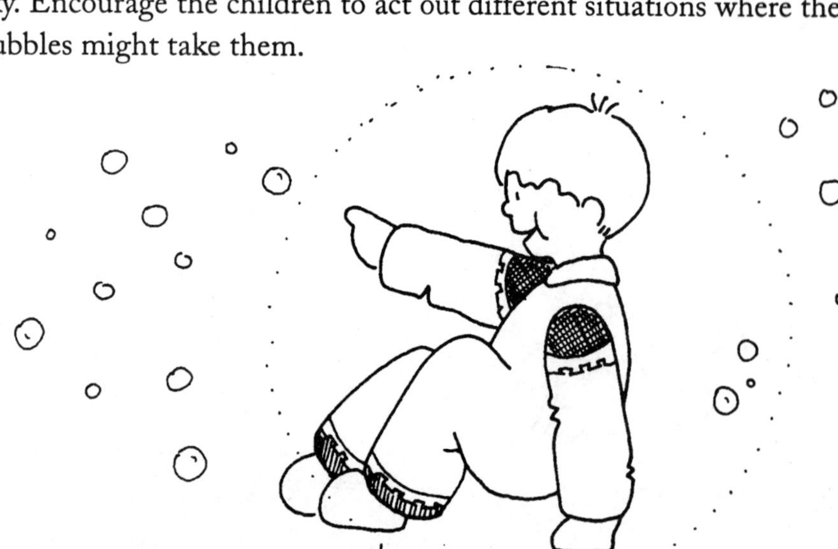

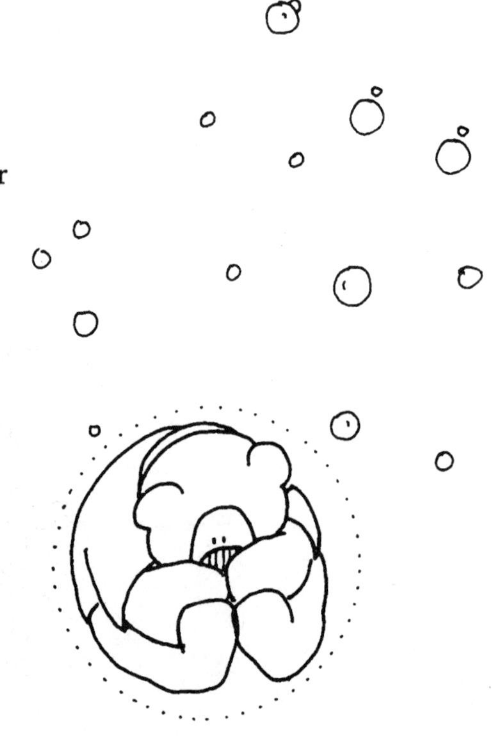

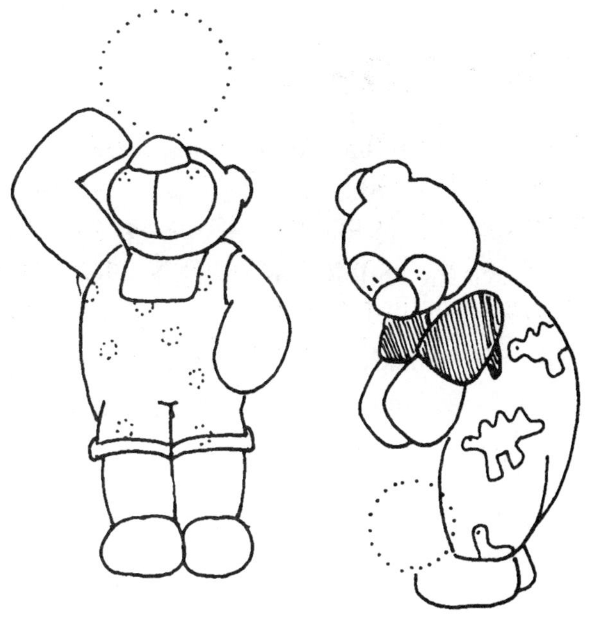

I Love Bubbles

Sung to: "The Battle Hymn of the Republic"

I blew a great big bubble and it landed on my nose.
(Point to nose.)

I blew a great big bubble and it landed on my toes.
(Point to toes.)

I blew a great big bubble and it landed on my knee.
(Point to knee.)

Oh, I love great big bubbles and they love me!
(Hug self.)

Jean Warren

My Bubble

Sung to: "My Bonnie Lies Over the Ocean"

My bubble flew over the ocean,
My bubble flew over the sea.
My bubble flew over the rainbow,
Oh, come back, my bubble, to me!

Come back, come back,
Oh, come back, my bubble, to me, to me.
Come back, come back,
Oh, come back, my bubble, to me!

Jean Warren

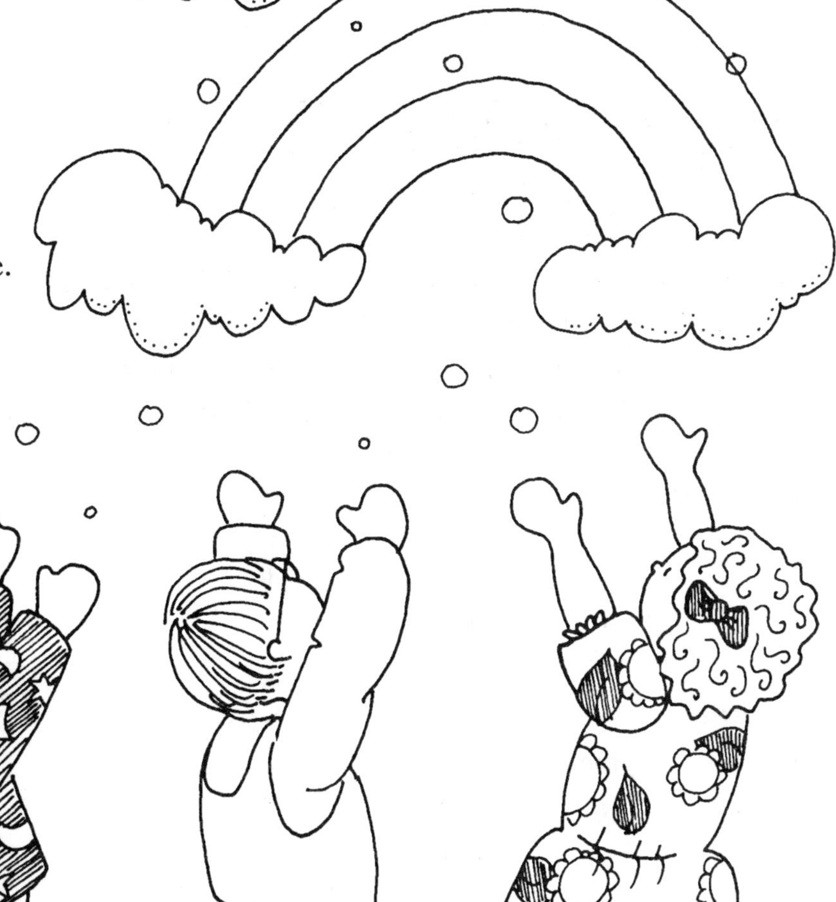

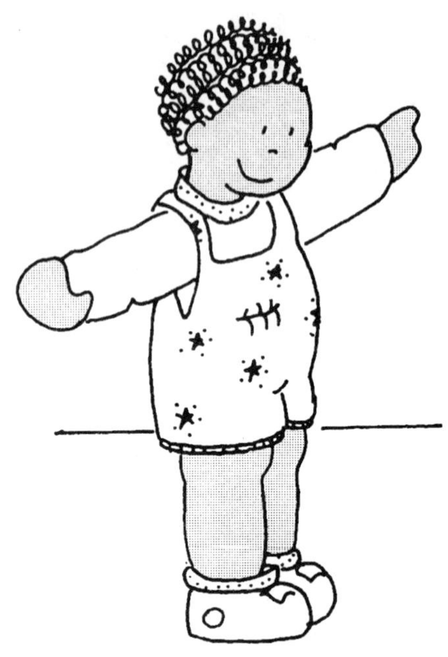

Ring Warm-Up

Tell your children that every circus has a ring in which the circus people perform their acts. Ask your children to help you make rings by holding out their arms and moving them in small circles, then bigger and bigger circles. Have the children spin their bodies in circles. Can they think of any other ways to make circles? When they have exhausted all their ideas for making circles by themselves, suggest that they join hands and step back to make one gigantic circle, or ring, for the circus.

Tightrope Walkers

Sung to: "Mary Had a Little Lamb"

Tightrope walkers balancing,
(Pretend to walk on tightrope.)
Balancing, balancing.
Tightrope walkers balancing
On a stretch of string.

Elephants are walking slow,
(Walk like an elephant.)
Walking slow, walking slow.
Elephants are walking slow,
In a line they go.

Bareback riders prance along,
(Prance around like horses.)
Prance along, prance along.
Bareback riders prance along
While they sing this song.

Jean Warren

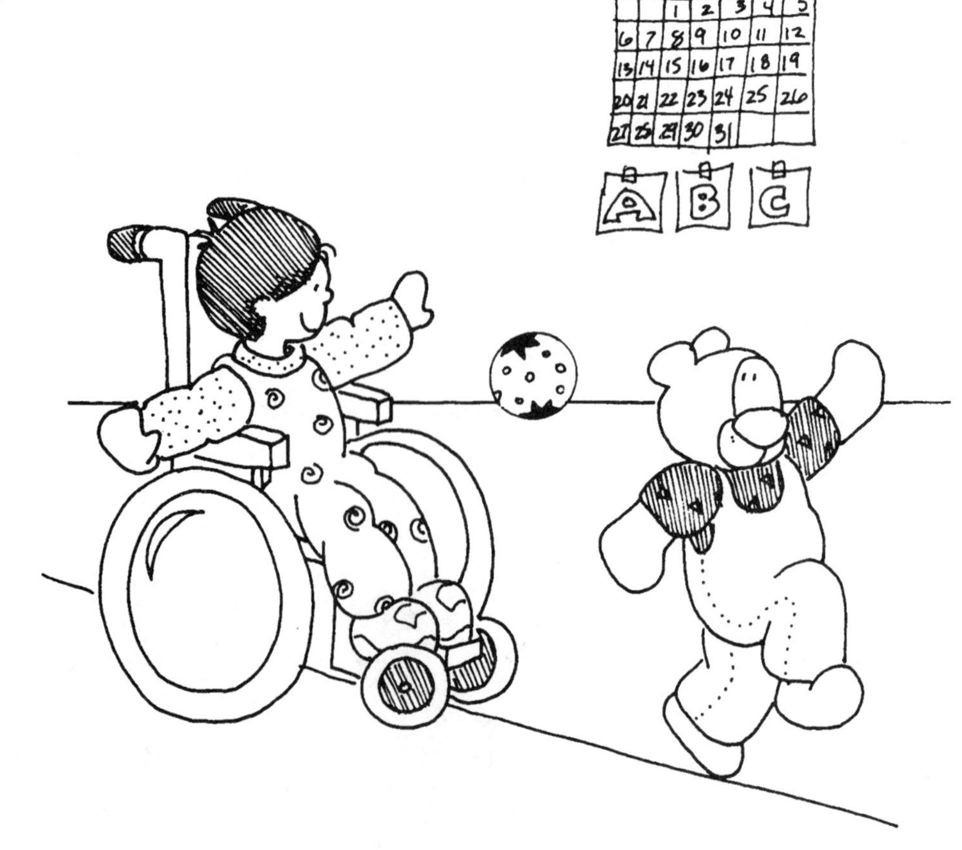

Circus Acts

Be the ringmaster of your children's circus and introduce the various circus acts that are being offered. Below are some performance possibilities.

- Have the children pretend to be prancing horses with decorated saddles, or the people who ride the horses and perform tricks on the saddles.
- Let the children pretend to be elephants and walk in a line, hooking their trunks (right hands) to the tails (left hands) of the elephants beside them. Or have the elephants perform by themselves, walking on a balance beam and swinging their long trunks.
- Encourage the children to pretend to walk the tightrope. Have them step very carefully on a straight line (a piece of yarn works well) with their arms held out on either side for balance.
- Let the children pretend to be acrobats and show off their somersaults, headstands, cartwheels, splits, or other tricks.
- Invite all the children to pretend to be clowns: Have them do silly tricks, such as running and falling, wiggling, and jumping.

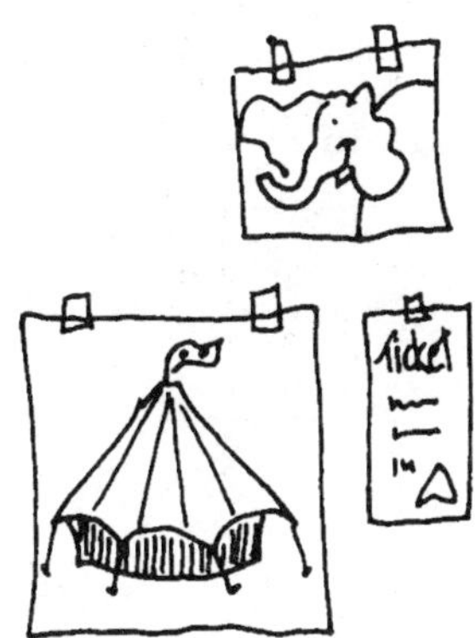

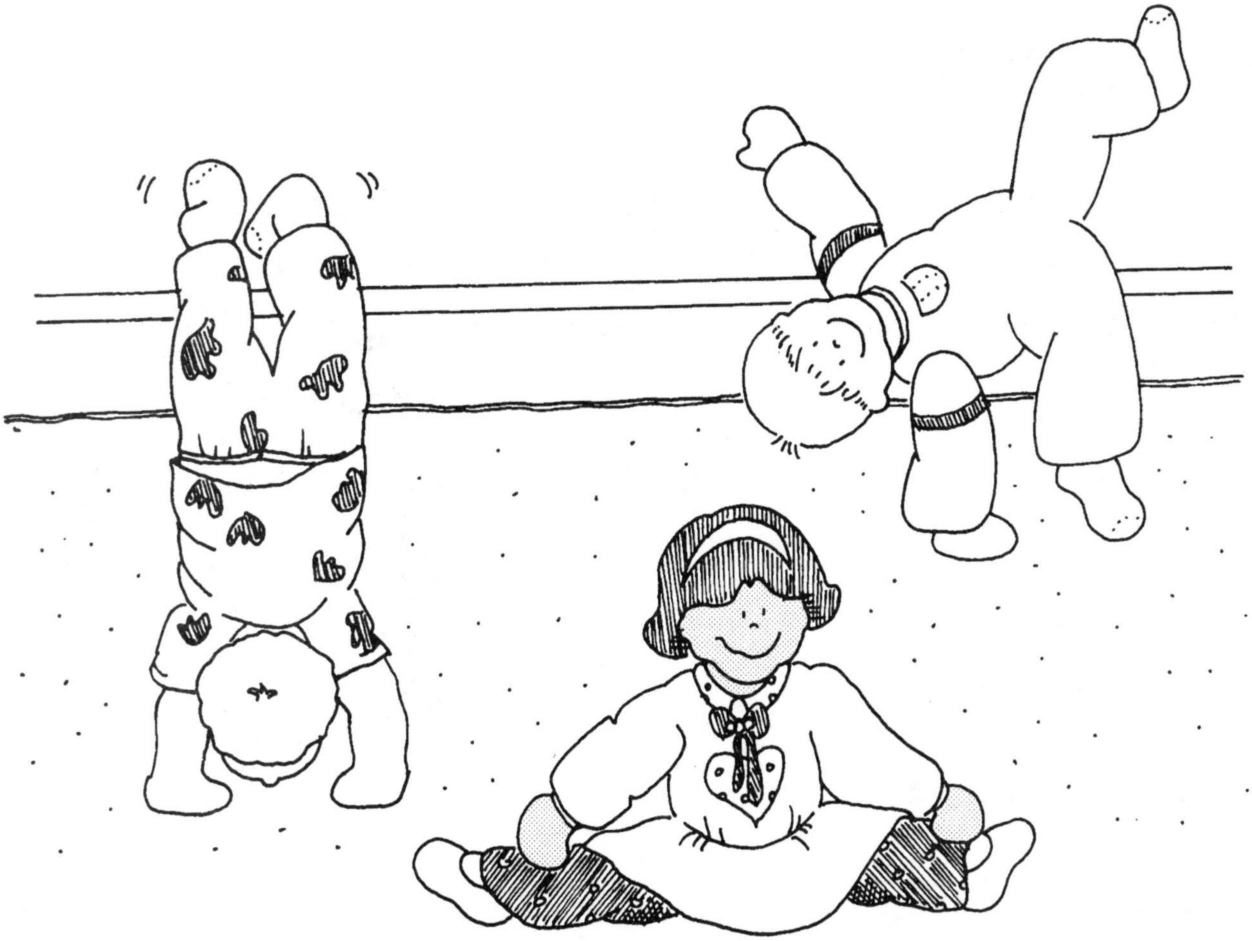

Balloon Warm-Up

Let your children observe you blow up a real balloon. How does the balloon look before it's blown up? Afterward? What happens when you let the air out? Have the children pretend to be limp balloons. As you pretend to blow them up, have them show you how they would expand, thrusting out their chests and opening their arms. After they have floated about lightly, let them "pop" each other with a finger so they deflate quickly. You may wish to have the children stand in a small circle before deflating, so they can rush backward without crashing into one another.

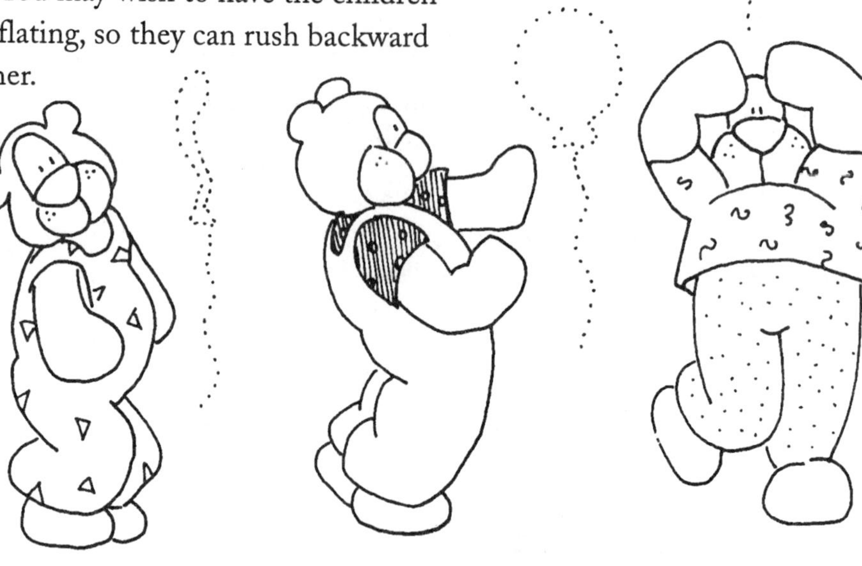

Balloon Poppers

Have the children pretend to blow up enough balloons to fill the room. Next, give each child a pretend pin to attach to a part of his or her body, such as a knee, toe, elbow, nose, or hip. Tell the children that they are now your Balloon Poppers. Have them reach high and low to pop all the pretend balloons you have floating in your room. Great exercise!

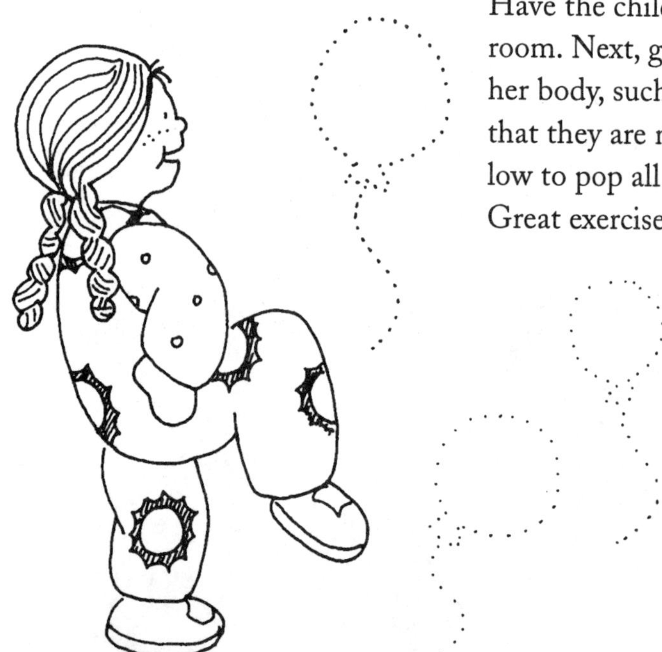

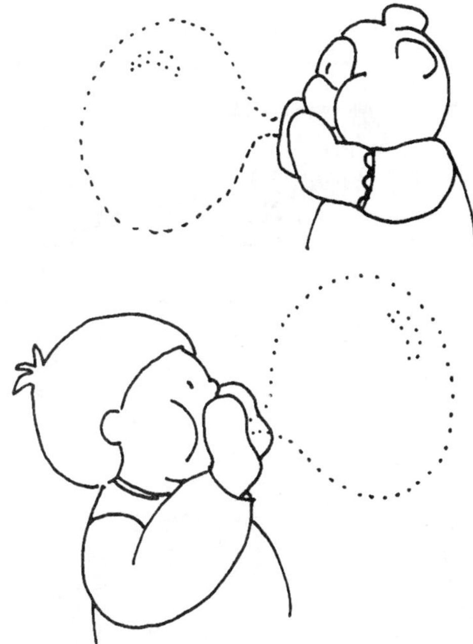

Blow Your Balloon

Have your children pretend to blow up balloons as you sing the following song. At the end of the song, have the children clap as their pretend balloons pop.

Sung to: "Row, Row, Row Your Boat"

Grab, grab, grab a balloon,
Give it a big blow.
The more you fill it up with air,
The bigger it will grow.

Blow, blow, blow your balloon,
Perhaps now you should stop.
For if you blow it up too much,
It will surely pop!

Jean Warren

A Little Balloon

A little balloon,
(Form circle with thumb and finger.)

A bigger balloon,
(Form circle with hands.)

A great big balloon I see.
(Form circle with arms.)

Now let's count them.

Are you ready?

One,
(Form circle with arms.)

Two,
(Form circle with hands.)

Three.
(Form circle with thumb and finger.)

Adapted Traditional

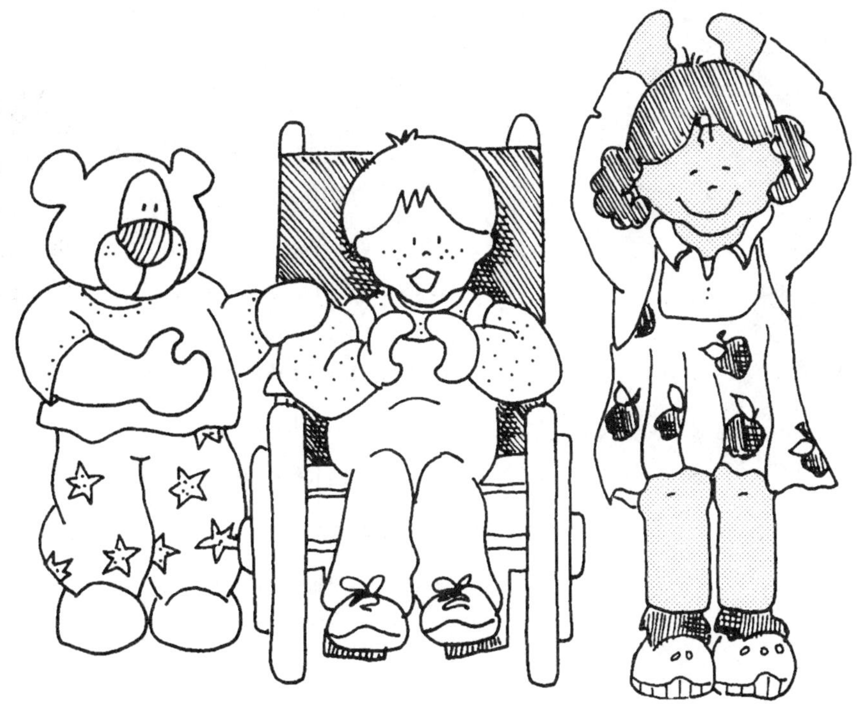

Bare Feet Warm-Up

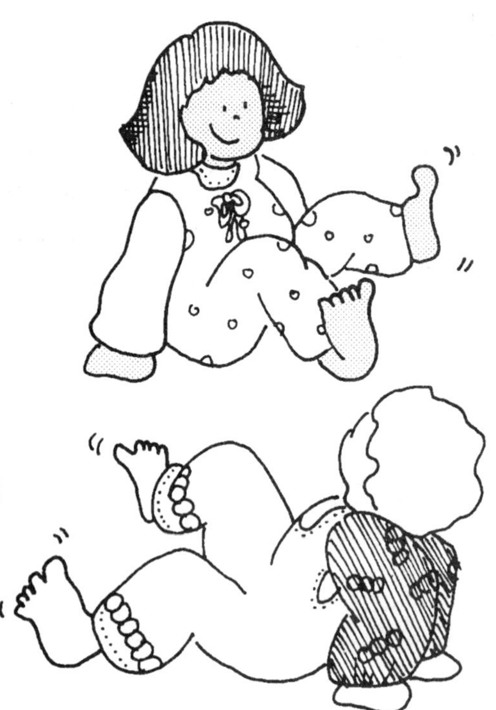

Children love to play in their bare feet, so this warm-up will be a natural. First, have the children remove their shoes and socks. Ask them to sit on the floor and concentrate on their feet, rubbing them against each other, wiggling their toes, knocking their big toes together, bobbing their heels, and bending their legs and stamping their feet.

Now, have them stand up and make their feet behave in different ways. Can their feet be quiet feet, sneaky feet, heavy feet, tiny feet, slow feet, clumsy feet? Have the children show you how their feet can walk, run, skip, march, and jump before they put their socks and shoes back on.

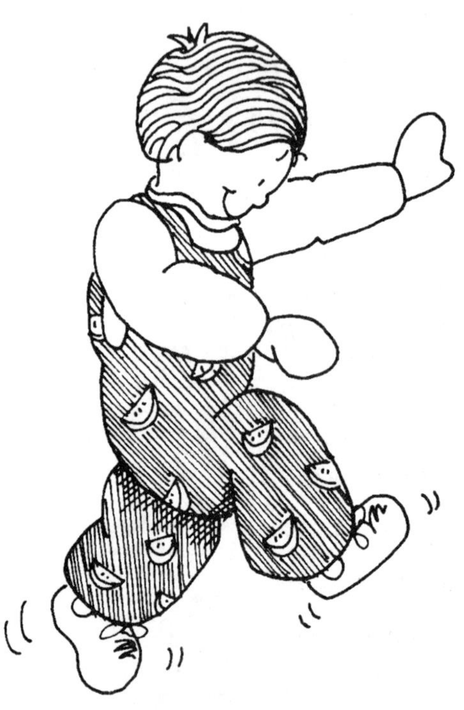

My Dancing Feet

Let your children pretend they have dancing feet while you sing the following song. Encourage them to dance as described in the song.

Sung to: "The Muffin Man"

Have you seen my dancing feet,
My dancing feet, my dancing feet?
Have you seen my dancing feet
As they dance on down the street?

Sometimes fast and sometimes slow,
Sometimes high and sometimes low—
Have you seen my dancing feet
As they dance on down the street?

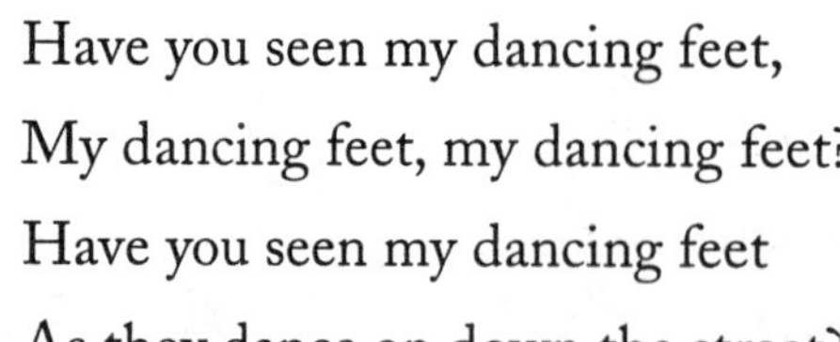

Additional verses: Have you seen my running feet; jumping feet; skipping feet; etc.

Jean Warren

Shoes

Ask your children to pretend to try on a variety of shoes and then show you how they would walk in them. For example, they could try on cowboy boots, ballet slippers, swim fins, ice skates, high heels, long clown shoes, galoshes, tap-dancing shoes, jogging shoes, basketball shoes, or an astronaut's moon-walking shoes.

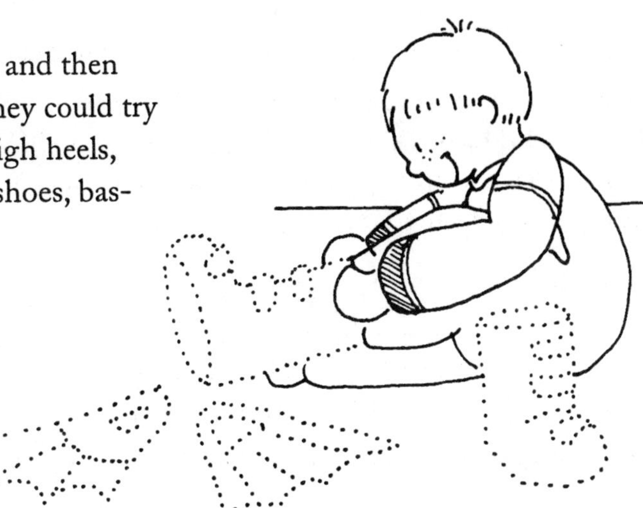

Magic Feet

Have your children act out the motions as you read the following rhyme.

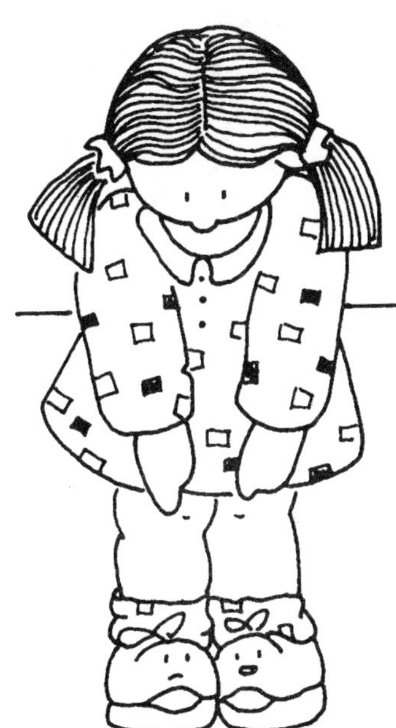

One day I found a pair of shoes
Out upon the walk.
They looked like any other shoes,
Except this pair could talk!

They told me they were special shoes
That I might wear that day.
I quickly slipped them on my feet
And headed out to play.

When I ran with all my friends,
My shoes went, oh, so fast.
I found myself out in the lead
Instead of near the last.

And when we started jumping
Over brooks and streams,
My feet just seemed to fly across
Like they do in dreams.

I wore my shoes while swimming
And swam across the lake.
I looked just like a motorboat—
I even left a wake.

Next, I tried some dancing,
The shoes were really neat.
They let me spin and leap and bend
And never miss a beat.

What a special day that was,
What a special treat
To have such fun at everything—
To have two magic feet!

Jean Warren

Travel Warm-Up

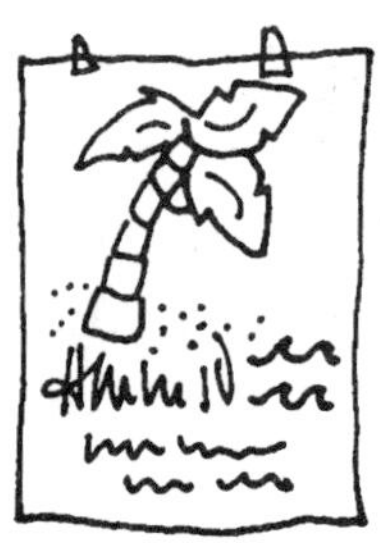

Tell the children that everyone is going on a trip together. Explain that you will be traveling in many different kinds of vehicles. Start your trip on bicycles. Show the children how to lie on their backs and pedal with their legs. While everyone is pedaling, ask the children to decide where they want to go.

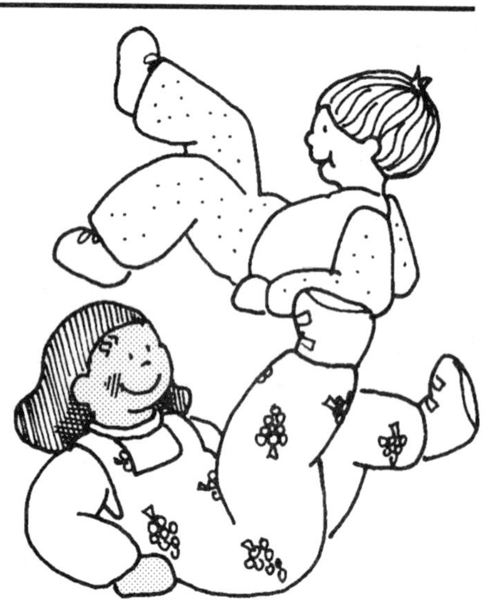

Make the sound of a train. Have the children jump off their bikes and hop aboard the train, making their arms move back and forth like the wheels. Form one long train by having the children line up and place their left hand on the shoulder of the person in front of them while continuing to rotate their right hand like train wheels.

When the children tire of the train, toot the whistle and say, "All out for ________!" (The destination they chose earlier.) For the return trip, recommend that they take a plane to make the trip short. After they have zoomed around the room, their radar signals working to prevent any midair collisions, let the children circle the airfield, lower their landing gear, and take turns landing.

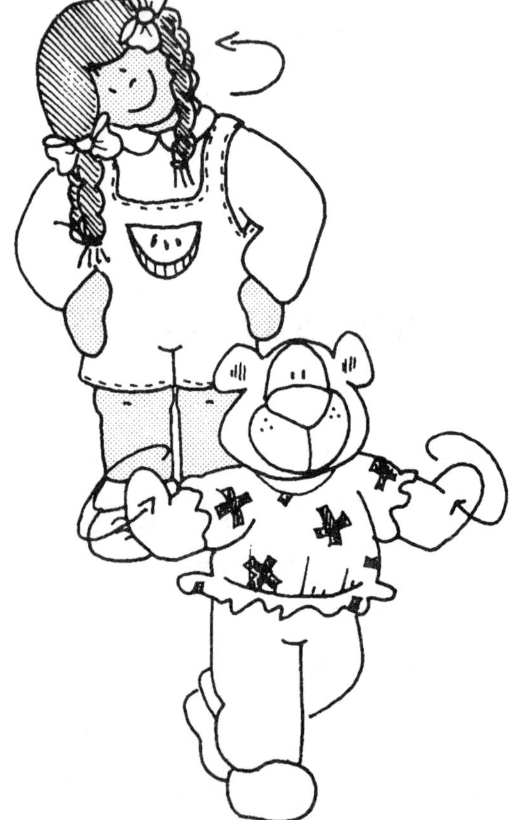

Body Wheels

How many ways can your children make wheels with their bodies? Can they make their heads turn like wheels? Their arms, hands, fingers, hips, legs, and feet? Can they make more than one body wheel move at a time? In different directions?

Have the children pair up and coordinate their bodies in some way to make a machine that runs on wheels—as many as possible. As a grand finale, have all the children come together and create one giant machine made up of many wheels and moving parts. Encourage the children to make all the wheels work together simultaneously. For a greater challenge, have one wheel begin turning, which then activates the wheel next to it, and so on until all the wheels are turning. As the last wheel turns, have the machine "Bong!" and wind down by having the wheels come to a slow stop in reverse order.

Off We Go

Let your children pretend to be the different vehicles as they are mentioned in the following song.

Sung to: "Frère Jacques"

Here's the train, here's the train.
All aboard, all aboard.
Chug-a-chug-a-choo-choo,
Chug-a-chug-a-choo-choo,
Off we go, off we go.

Here's the airplane, here's the airplane.
All aboard, all aboard.
Chug-a-chug-a-zoom-zoom,
Chug-a-chug-a-zoom, zoom,
Off we go, off we go.

Here's the boat, here's the boat.
All aboard, all aboard.
Chug-a-chug-a-toot-toot,
Chug-a-chug-a-toot-toot,
Off we go, off we go.

Jean Warren

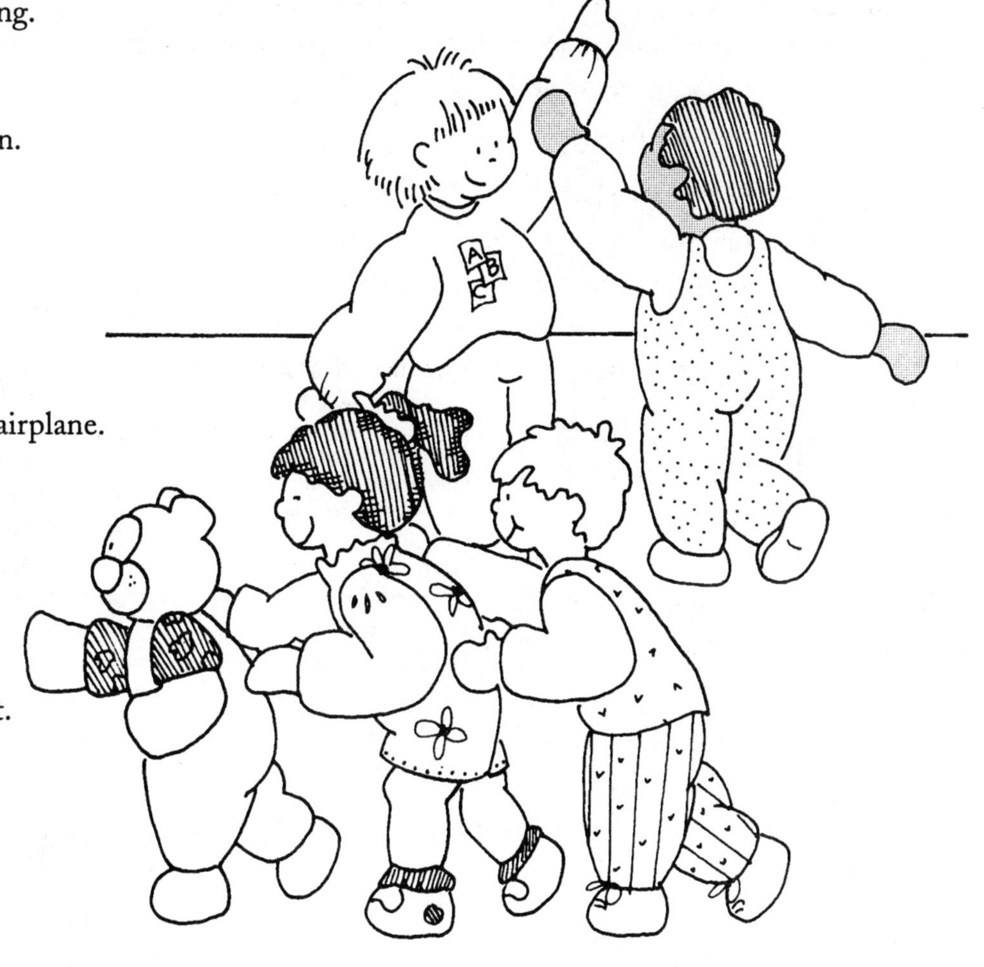

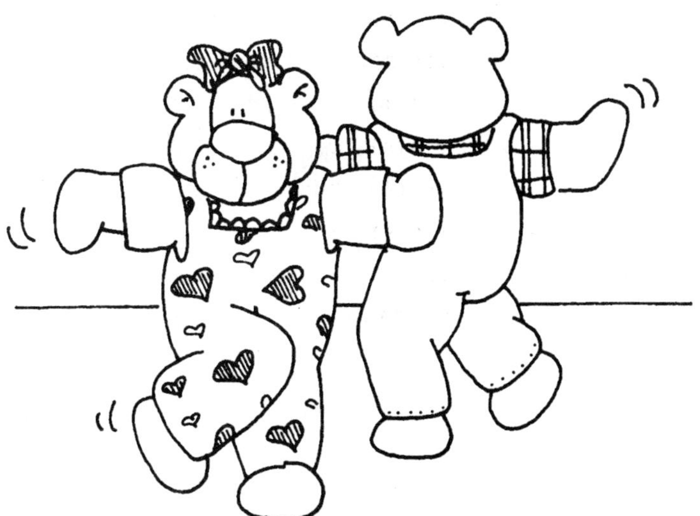

Wheels Turning

Sung to: "Frère Jacques"

I am moving, I am moving.
See me turn, see me turn.
First I turn one way,
Then I turn the other way.
See me turn, see me turn.

Jean Warren

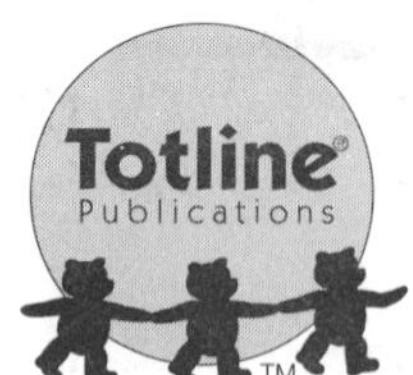

Teacher Resources

from Totline® Publications

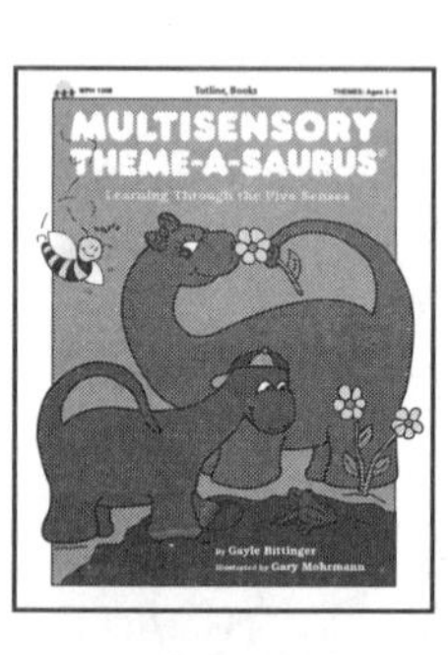

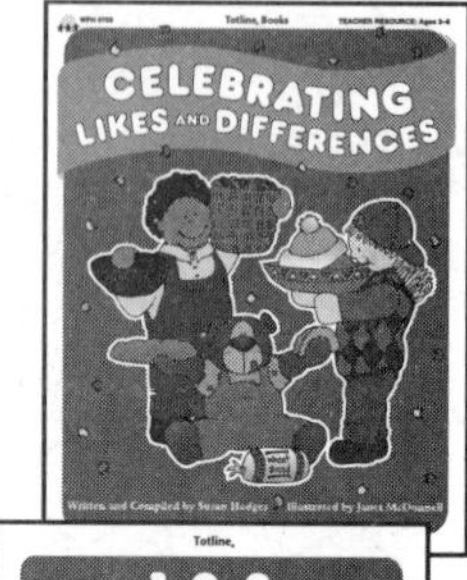

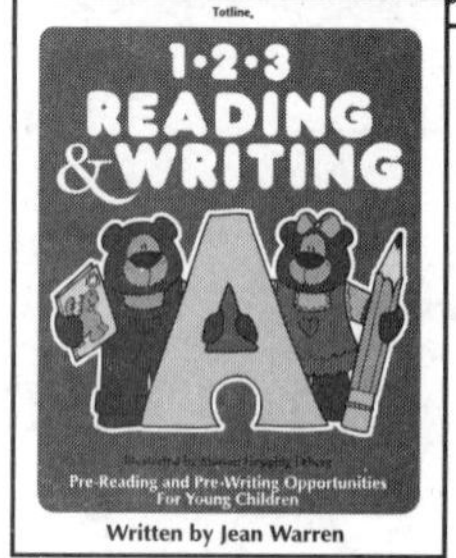

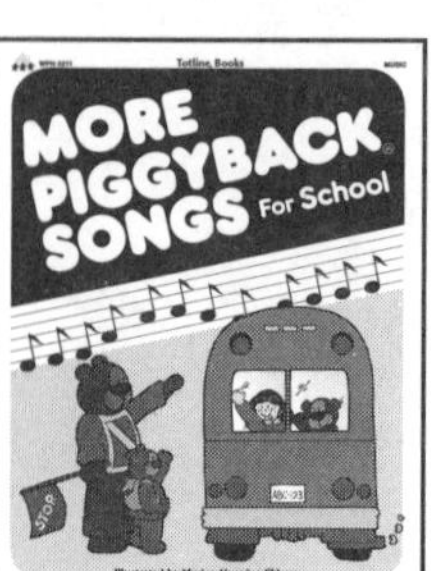

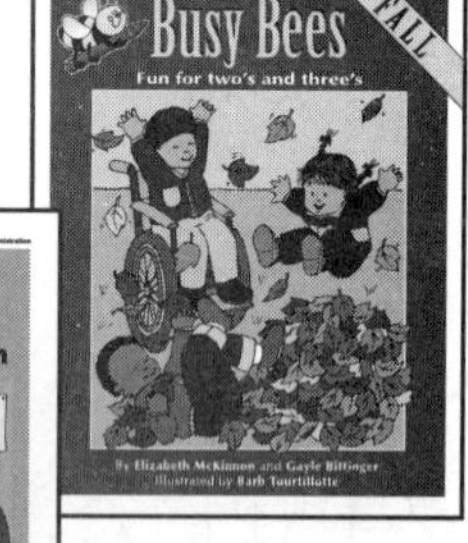

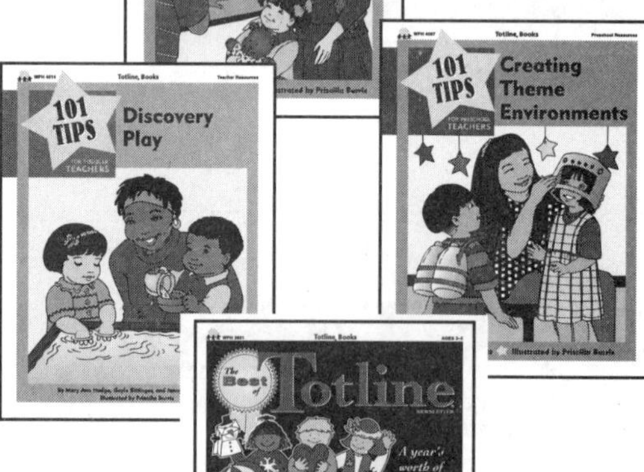

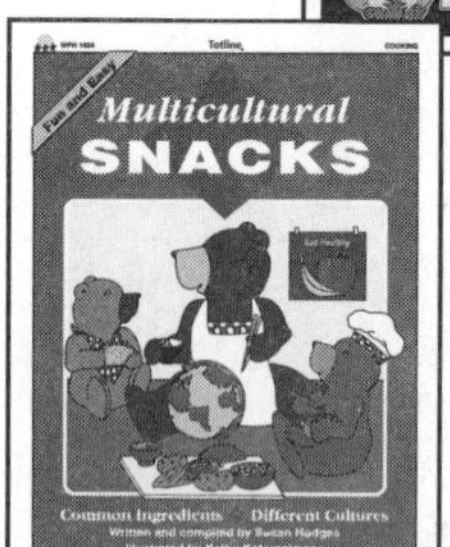

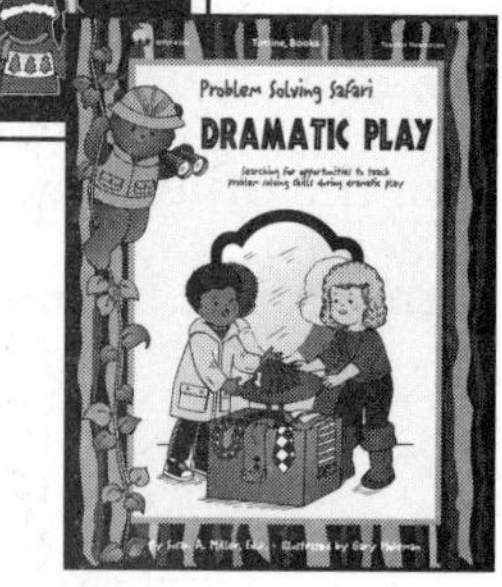

Celebrations

Easy, practical ideas for celebrating holidays and special days around the world. Plus ideas for making ordinary days special.

Celebrating Likes and Differences
Small World Celebrations
Special Day Celebrations
Great Big Holiday Celebrations

Theme-A-Saurus®

Classroom-tested, around-the-curriculum activities organized into imaginative units. Great for implementing a child-directed program.

Multisensory Theme-A-Saurus
Theme-A-Saurus
Theme-A-Saurus II
Toddler Theme-A-Saurus
Alphabet Theme-A-Saurus
Nursery Rhyme Theme-A-Saurus
Storytime Theme-A-Saurus

1•2•3 Series

Open-ended, age-appropriate, cooperative, and no-lose experiences for working with preschool children.

1•2•3 Art
1•2•3 Games
1•2•3 Colors
1•2•3 Puppets
1•2•3 Reading & Writing
1•2•3 Rhymes, Stories & Songs
1•2•3 Math
1•2•3 Science
1•2•3 Shapes

Snacks Series

Easy, educational recipes for healthy eating and expanded learning.

Super Snacks
Healthy Snacks
Teaching Snacks
Multicultural Snacks

Piggyback® Songs

New songs sung to the tunes of childhood favorites. No music to read! Easy for adults and children to learn. Chorded for guitar or autoharp.

Piggyback Songs
More Piggyback Songs
Piggyback Songs for Infants & Toddlers
Piggyback Songs in Praise of God
Piggyback Songs in Praise of Jesus
Holiday Piggyback Songs
Animal Piggyback Songs
Piggyback Songs for School
Piggyback Songs to Sign
Spanish Piggyback Songs
More Piggyback Songs for School

Busy Bees

These seasonal books help two- and three-year-olds discover the world around them through their senses. Each book includes fun activity and learning ideas, songs, snack ideas, and more!

Busy Bees—SPRING
Busy Bees—SUMMER
Busy Bees—FALL
Busy Bees—WINTER

101 Tips for Directors

Great ideas for managing a preschool or daycare. These hassle-free, handy hints are a great help.

Staff and Parent Self-Esteem
Parent Communication
Health and Safety
Marketing Your Center
Resources for You and Your Center
Child Development Training

101 Tips for Toddler Teachers

Designed for adults who work with toddlers.

Classroom Management
Discovery Play
Dramatic Play
Large Motor Play
Small Motor Play
Word Play

101 Tips for Preschool Teachers

Valuable, fresh ideas for adults who work with young children.

Creating Theme Environments
Encouraging Creativity
Developing Motor Skills
Developing Language Skills
Teaching Basic Concepts
Spicing Up Learning Centers

Problem Solving Safari

This unique series teaches teachers to help children problem-solve and think for themselves. Each book includes scenarios from children's real play and possible solutions.

Problem Solving Safari—Art
Problem Solving Safari—Blocks
Problem Solving Safari—Dramatic Play
Problem Solving Safari—Manipulatives
Problem Solving Safari—Outdoors
Problem Solving Safari—Science

The Best of Totline® Series

Collections of some of the finest, most useful material published in *Totline Magazine* over the years.

The Best of Totline
The Best of Totline Parent Flyers

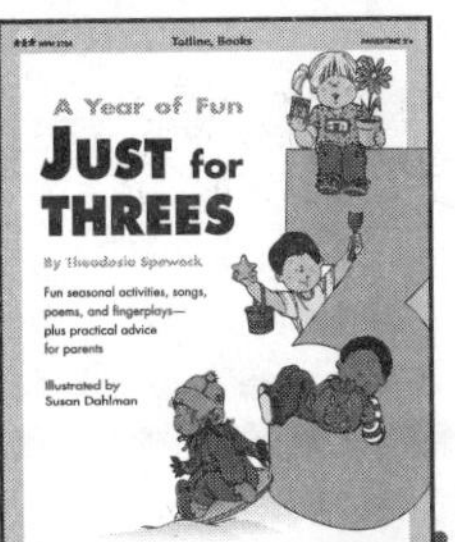

Early Learning at its Best

For parents and children: books, posters, puzzles and more from Totline® Publications

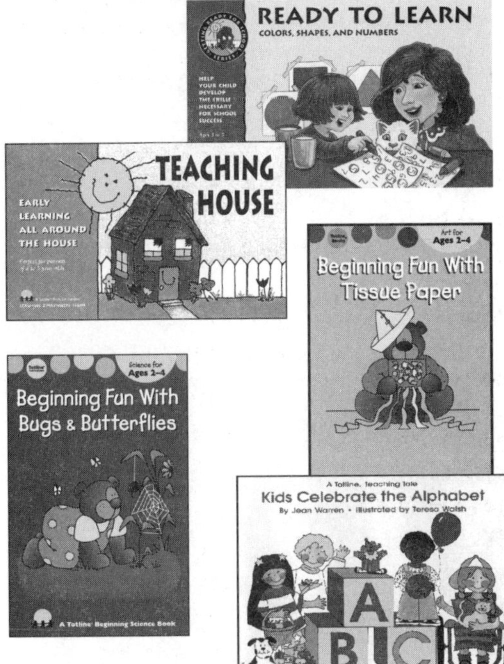

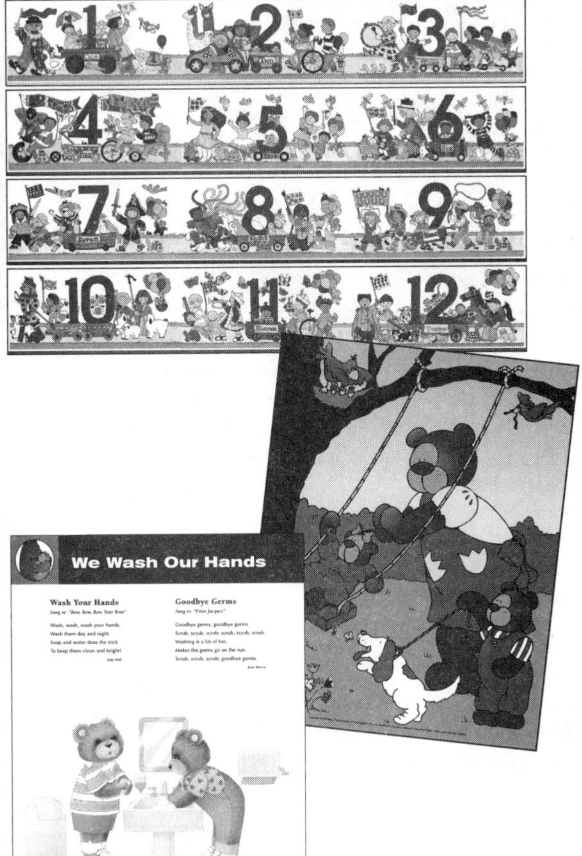

A Year of Fun

Age-specific books detailing how young children grow and change and what parents can do to lay a strong foundation for later learning.

Just for Babies
Just for Ones
Just for Twos
Just for Threes
Just for Fours
Just for Fives

Getting Ready for School

Fun, easy-to-follow ideas for developing essential skills that preschoolers need before they can successfully achieve higher levels of learning.

Ready to Learn Colors, Shapes, and Numbers
Ready to Write and Develop Motor Skills
Ready to Read
Ready to Communicate
Ready to Listen and Explore the Senses

Learning Everywhere

Teaches parents to become aware of the everyday opportunities for teaching their children about language, art, science, math, problem solving, self-esteem, and more!

Teaching House
Teaching Town
Teaching Trips

Beginning Fun With Art

Introduce young children to the fun of art while developing coordination skills and building self-confidence.

Craft Sticks • Crayons • Felt
Glue • Paint • Paper Shapes
Modeling Dough • Yarn
Tissue Paper • Scissors
Rubber Stamps • Stickers

Beginning Fun With Science

Make science fun with these quick, safe, easy-to-do activities that lead to discovery and spark the imagination.

Bugs & Butterflies
Plants & Flowers
Magnets
Rainbows & Colors
Sand & Shells
Water & Bubbles

Teaching Tales

Each of these children's books includes a delightful story plus related activity ideas that expand on the story's theme.

Kids Celebrate the Alphabet
Kids Celebrate Numbers
Ellie the Evergreen
The Wishing Fish
The Bear and the Mountain
Huff and Puff's Snowy Day
Huff and Puff on Groundhog Day
Huff and Puff's Hawaiian Rainbow
Huff and Puff Go to Camp
Huff and Puff on Fourth of July
Huff and Puff Around the World
Huff and Puff Go to School
Huff and Puff on Halloween
Huff and Puff on Thanksgiving
Huff and Puff's Foggy Christmas

Learning Puzzles

Designed to challenge as children grow. Each giant floor puzzle offers learning opportunities, plus teaches basic matching and thinking skills.

Kids Celebrate Numbers Beginning Floor Puzzle
Kids Celebrate the Alphabet Beginning Floor Puzzle
Bear Hugs 4-in-1 Puzzle Set
Busy Bees 4-in-1 Puzzle Set

Two-Sided Circle Puzzles

Double-sided, giant floor puzzles designed in a circle with cutout pieces for extra learning and fun.

Underwater Adventure
African Adventure

Work and Play Together Posters

A colorful collection of cuddly bear posters showing adult and children bears playing and working together. Each 17"x 22".

We Build Together
We Cook Together
We Play Together
We Read Together
We Sing Together
We Work Together

Bear Hugs® Sing-Along Health Posters

Encourage young children to develop good health habits with these posters. Additional learning activities on back!

We Brush Our Teeth
We Can Exercise
We Cover our Coughs and Sneezes
We Eat Good Food
We Get Our Rest
We Wash Our Hands

Totline products are available at fine parent and teacher stores.

For the dealer nearest you, call 1-800-421-5565.

If you like Totline® Books,

You'll love Totline® Magazine!

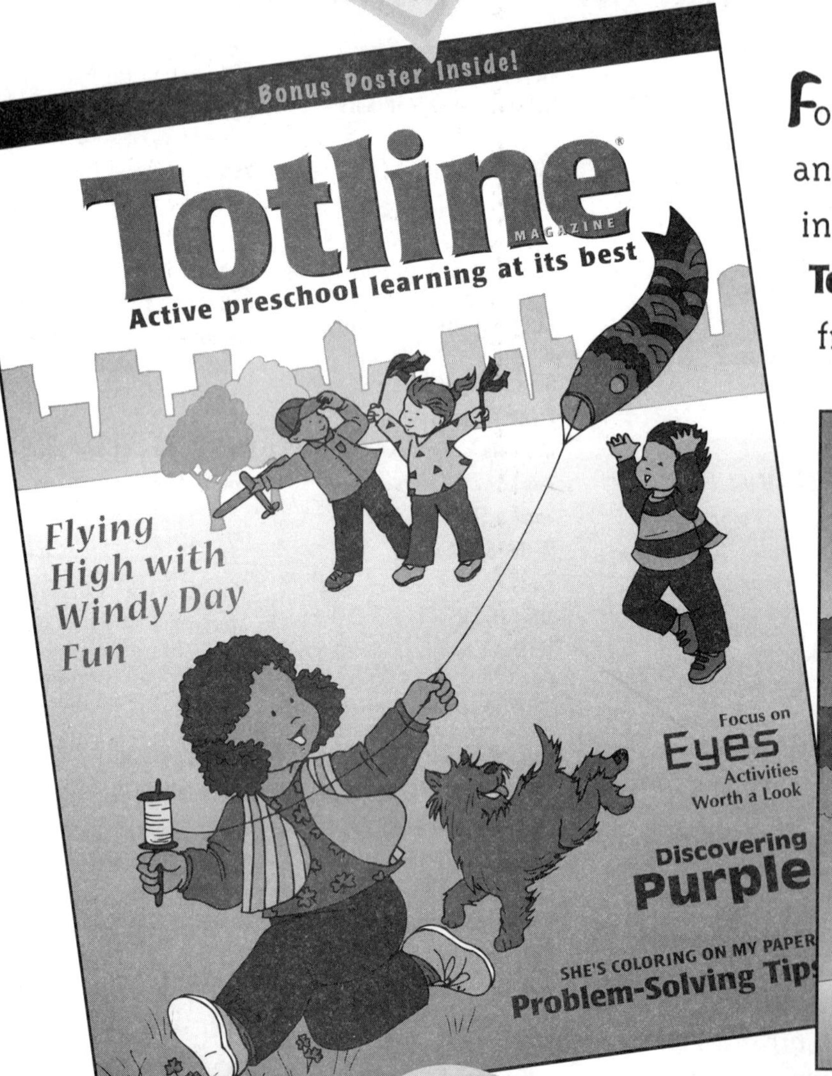

For fresh ideas that challenge and engage young children in active learning, reach for **Totline® Magazine**—Proven ideas from innovative teachers!

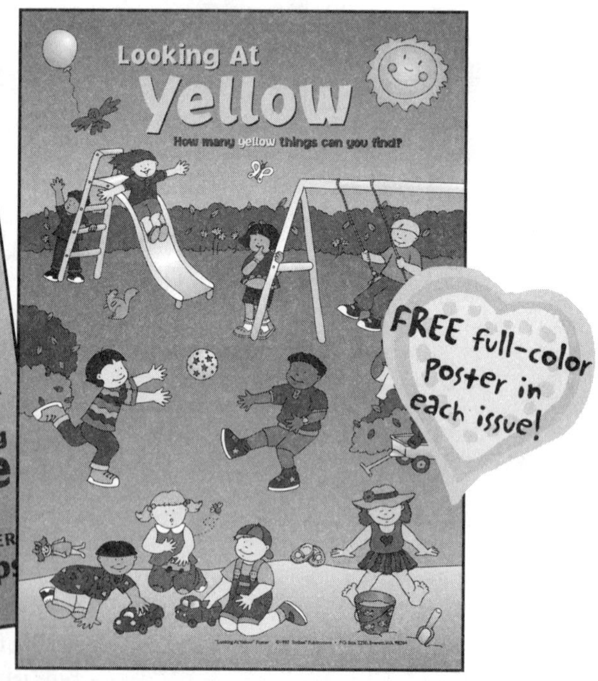

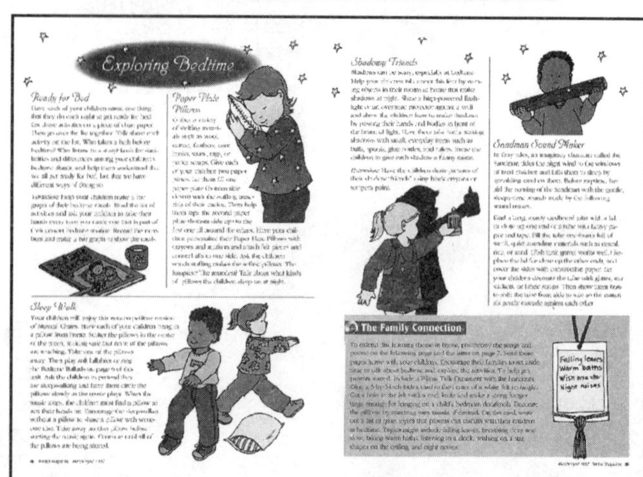

Exploring Bedtime

Ready for Bed

Paper Plate Pillows

Shadowy Friends

Sandman Sound Maker

Sleep Walk

The Family Connection

Each issue includes

- Seasonal learning themes
- Stories, songs, and rhymes
- Open-ended art projects
- Science explorations
- Reproducible parent pages
- Ready-made teaching materials
- Activities just for toddlers
- Reproducible healthy snack recipes

Receive a FREE copy of Totline® Magazine by calling 800-609-1724 for subscription information.